RECENT ADVANCES IN HEMATOLOGY RESEARCH

CORD BLOOD

BANKS AND BANKING, ETHICAL ISSUES AND RISKS/BENEFITS

Recent Advances in Hematology Research

Additional books in this series can be found on Nova's website under the Series tab.

Additional e-books in this series can be found on Nova's website under the e-book tab.

Public Health in the 21st Century

Additional books in this series can be found on Nova's website under the Series tab.

Additional e-books in this series can be found on Nova's website under the e-book tab.

RECENT ADVANCES IN HEMATOLOGY RESEARCH

CORD BLOOD

BANKS AND BANKING, ETHICAL ISSUES AND RISKS/BENEFITS

LISANDRA VANOSTRAND
EDITOR

New York

For permission to use material from this book please contact us:
Telephone 631-231-7269; Fax 631-231-8175
Web Site: http://www.novapublishers.com

Library of Congress Cataloging-in-Publication Data

ISBN: 978-1-62618-072-7
Library of Congress Control Number: 2013931036

Published by Nova Science Publishers, Inc. † New York

Contents

Preface

In this book, the authors discuss cord blood banks and banking, the ethical issues involved and the risks and benefits. Topics include the virological risks and benefits of cord blood banking; mesenchymal stem cells and their role in regenerative medicine applications; osteogenic potential of human umbilical cord-derived mesenchymal stromal cells; public versus private cord blood banking; CCR5 deficient cord blood as a means of treatment for HIV-1 infection; and the therapeutic use of umbilical cord blood.

Chapter 1 - The risks of the reactivation of latently carried maternal viruses during pregnancy and the transfer of primary maternal viral infections to fetus due to the maternal immunomodulation may also affect the safety of the umbilical cord blood banking. Microchymerism, transcytosis, transfer of virus-immunoglobulin complexes and replication of viruses in placental and fetal cells are the mechanisms of the maternal-fetal transfer of viruses. Very few virus harbouring cells in the cord blood preparations might endanger the health of transplant recipients. Very few cells with latent viruses can be amplified and released during the *in vitro* expansion of the pluripotent umbilical cord blood cell (UCB) populations.

There is a consensus in the literature, that serology only cannot be used for the detection of contaminating viruses. Real time PCR, and or microchips under development seem to be the best, and quickest methodology for this purpose. It seems to be necessary to broaden the spectrum of viruses to be screened at present. In case the microchip technology will be available, certain interleukins, tumor necrosis factors and interferons might be also included into the preliminary testing. Micro-RNA and or exosome specific molecules might be considered for preliminary testing, since these are indirect markers of virus infections. Viral transactivator proteins TAT, NEF and TAX proteins of HIV1-

2 and HTLV 1-4 human retroviruses and HBeAg of hepatitis B virus can pass the placenta and modify cellular function of fetal cells even in the absence of the viruses themselves.

In case the microchip technologies will be routinly introduced, these molecules and also certain lectins (CD161) should be added to the list of viral products, to be tested. The methodology of the UCB control and that of the post-transplantation surveillance has to be completely different.

Contamination with viruses is not always a contraindication to preserve samples. In case appropriate active vaccination for the prevention of the disease or specific chemotherapy are available. This is especially true for enteroviruses, orthomyxoviruses etc. preventable simply by humoral immunity. Herpesviruses, papillomaviruses, hepatitis B virus, and viruses such as torque teno anellovirus, GB-C/HGV flavivirus, which had not been associated with clinical illnesses.

Transplacental transport of IgG might be useful, but the presence of viruses may reduce the pluripotency of fetal cell clones, certain lymphocyte receptor populations can be eliminated whithout any remarkable signs. The transfer of anti-idiotypes may induce fetal IgM synthesis in the second half of pregnancy, or eliminate certain clones of germline subgroups of B, NK, T and dendritic cells during the first half of pregnancy.

Maternal virus infections might result fetal modifications (interleukins, exosomes, tumor necrosis factors, interferons) even in the absence of the infection of the fetuses. Maternal-fetal virus transmission was shown to increase from the first trimester untill delivery, the fetal damage, however, is decreasing with time.

The perspectives of the umbilical cord blood transplantation are exponencially improving with the devlopment of molecular and recombination technologies.

Chapter 2 – *Introduction:* Current treatments for various degenerative disorders rely on surgical interventions and drugs that modulate the system, but these have their own limitations when it comes to regeneration of damaged tissues and cells. To address this shortcoming, cell-based therapies are gaining importance. Adult stem cells have generated great amount of interest amongst the scientific community for their potential therapeutic applications for unmet medical needs. Haematopoietic stem cells and MSCs are the two widely studied and characterized adult stem cells. Mesenchymal stem cells as a choice for cell-based therapies in regenerative medicine are becoming very clear.

Sources for MSCs: Currently, BM represents the main source of MSCs for both experimental and clinical studies, but with limitations. Bone marrow -

mesenchymal stem cells have been used in several clinical trials in various domains, such as, cardiology, neurology, and so on, with its limitations in the autologous settings, as it represents 0.01-0.001% of the nucleated cells in the adult human marrow. Hence, to overcome these limitations there is a need for an alternative source, which is easily available, noncontroversial, and could generate a higher number of MSCs. Therefore, the search for alternative sources of MSCs is of significant value. Of these different sources, human umbilical cord blood, cord tissue and adipose tissue could successfully replace BM as a source for MSCs.

Characterization of MSCs: MSCs, as defined by the International Society for Cellular Therapy (ISCT), are multipotent, spindle like plastic adherent cells capable of self-renewal and possess the ability to differentiate *in vitro* to bone, cartilage and adipose tissues. Phenotypic characterization studies of MSCs have shown that these cells express CD73, CD105, CD90, CD29 and CD44 cell surface antigens, and are negative for CD34, CD45, CD31, CD14, human leukocyte antigen (HLA)-class II antigens and von Willebrand factor. Recently some interesting molecules were described which may be useful to identify MSC (sub) populations (CD271, GD2, CD49a, W7C5, W8B2, C15, CDCP1, CD340, CD349, SSEA1/4). However, a distinct exclusively MSC-restricted marker has yet to be identified.

Differentiation to Mesodermal, Ectodermal and Endodermal Lineages: In vitro differentiation studies have shown that MSCs could differentiate to additional cell types encompassing mesodermal (myocytes and tendon), as well as cells of ectodermal (neurons) and endodermal (hepatocytes, pancreatic) lineages. Various studies induced MSC differentiation into neurons and glial cells. After *in vitro* neural differentiation cells demonstrated an assortment of neuronal and glial markers, such as neuronspecific enolase (NSE), neuronal nuclear antigen (NeuN), neurofilament M (NF-M), tau, glial fibrillary acidic protein (GFAP) and adopted neuronal and glial morphology. Rat MSC were stimulated to differentiate into cells with hepatocyte-like phenotypes after treatment with HGF.

Preclinical Studies: Animal studies have provided a useful tool for defining a number of diverse potential applications for MSCs. Recent studies have shown that BMMSCs improve neurological deficits when transplanted into animal models of neurological disorders. Studies in rodents suggest a broad initial biodistribution followed by a limited capacity for sustained engraftment. In fetal sheep, MSCs undergo a wide tissue distribution and can differentiate into multiple mesenchymal tissues following peritoneal implantation.It has been demonstrated that cultured mesenchymal cells could home to the bone marrow in non-human primates.

Immunological aspects of MSCs: First, the MSCs have the ability to repopulate the damaged host tissue for repair and restoration and second, these cells exert their immunomodulatory and immunosuppressive properties to survive in allogeneic hosts. *In vivo* observations after administration of MSC, like improvement of the outcome after allogeneic transplantations by promotion of hematopoietic engraftment and amelioration of graftversus- host disease as well as the amelioration of inflammatory response and improved clinical course in experimental allergic encephalomyelitis are impressive proofs for the immunomodulatory properties of MSC. Experimental data suggest that both cell surface molecules and soluble factors regulate the hypoimmunogenic, anti-inflammatory and anti-proliferative properties of MSCs.

Clinical Applications: In vivo transplantation of undifferentiated MSCs from various tissues, predominantly from the bone marrow, has shown therapeutic efficacy in experimental models of human diseases. All these properties of MSCs, along with their non-tumorigenic nature, have made them attractive candidate for human clinical use, mainly in autologous cell transplantation to treat degenerative diseases. MSCs are currently studied as treatment for inflammatory diseases such as graft-versus host--disease, but also as treatment for myocardial infarct and solid organ transplantation.

Conclusion: MSCs can be differentiated into distinct different skeletal tissues both in *vitro* and *in vivo*. This versatile and tunable differentiation potential of MSCs in conjunction with their ability to secrete various trophic factors and modulate the recipient's immune system makes them a promising cell source in regenerative medicine. Most of the research has been done in the last decade focusing on characterizing MSCs and understanding their differentiation potential. However, the complex mechanisms and pathways with which MSCs supports repair are far from fully understood.Their immunosuppressive capabilities without evidence of immunosuppressive toxicity at a global level define their application in the treatment of diseases in which the pathogenesis involves uncontrolled activity of the immune system.

Chapter 3 - The presence of umbilical cord-derived mesenchymal stem cells has been reported. In the present study, the authors used autoserum derived from the umbilical cord blood (UCB) of neonates in an attempt to examine the osteoblastic differentiation potential of umbilical cord-derived mesenchymal stromal cells (UC-MSCs) in nude mice.

UCB, hydroxyapatite, and rhBMP were used as the supply source of autologous serum, scaffold, and osteoinductive growth factor, respectively. MSCs, obtained from Wharton jelly and cultured for 3 to 4 weeks to induce their differentiation into osteoblasts, were implanted subcutaneously into the dorsum of male nude mice for 6 weeks before the assessment by real-time reverse transcriptase polymerase chain reaction of osteoblast marker expression.

UCB-derived autologous serum was sufficient for the culture and implantation of UC-MSCs. The osteoblastic differentiation potential of UC-MSCs was demonstrated in nude mice by the conduct of immunohistochemical staining and by the investigation of osteoblast marker expression. The authors' results suggest the osteogenic potential of UC-MSCs and provide basic evidence for the realization of regenerative medicine using materials obtained from UC and UCB.

Chapter 4 - This chapter seeks to identify some ethical issues associated with public and private cord blood banks. After a brief report on existing cord blood banks worldwide, it aims to stimulate ethical reflections about allogenic versus autologous cord blood transplants. Whereas allogenic (related and unrelated) transplantation of umbilical cord blood is scientifically recognized as a proven treatment for several diseases affecting both children and adults, private cord blood banks promote a service – namely, the storage of the newborn cord blood for autologous transplant – which is not presently supported by clinical evidence. This raises critical issues in ethical terms ranging from the legitimacy of the informed consent process to the breach of the principle of justice requiring a fair distribution of available cord blood units among patients who need a cord blood transplant.

Chapter 5 - Infection with the human immunodeficiency virus type 1 (HIV-1) causes a continuous decrease of T-cells ending in the acquired immune deficiency syndrome (AIDS). HIV-1 requires the presence of a CD4 receptor and a chemokine receptor, namely CCR5. The most encouraging method of interrupting the interaction of the viral surface glycoprotein gp120 with this coreceptor involves the replacement of wild-type CCR5 with a truncated form of the receptor encoded by a 32 base-pair deletion (CCR5-delta32) in the CCR5 gene. Recently, the successful stem cell transplantation (SCT) of an HIV-1-infected patient suffering from acute myeloid leukemia, applying homozygous CCR5-delta32 donor cells has been reported. These hematopoietic progenitor cells engrafted, proliferated, and differentiated to produce mature myeloid and lymphoid cells that were highly resistant to HIV-1 infection. Currently, over 5 years after the transplantation and in the absence of any antiretroviral treatment, no plasma viral load or proviral DNA are detectable in peripheral blood cells and certain tissue samples in this patient.

However, current attempts to repeat this approach failed due to the availability of matching CCR5 negative stem cell donors. To increase the probability in finding a matching donor Stemcyte and other facilities, built up databases with pretested umbilical cord blood units (UCB), genotyped for the CCR5-delta32 deletion. An international collaboration of HIV researches and transplant centers initiated in 2012 an initiative to carry on the idea of the use of UCB from CCR5-delta32 homozygous donors in patients with HIV requiring SCT.

Chapter 6 - Umbilical cord blood (UCB) is an alternative source to bone marrow or peripheral blood to obtain functional hematopoietic stem cells (HSCs) for transplantation to reconstitute the blood and immune system after myeloablative or radiation therapy for numerous malignant and nonmalignant conditions. Since the world's first UCB transplant was performed in 1988, over 10,000 UCB transplants have been conducted worldwide. The use of UCB is now expected to grow not only because more UCB units are available for traditional hematopoietic transplantation but also because new stem cell therapies such as regenerative medicine have emerged into clinical applications.

This chapter summarizes UCB biology, storage methods for UCB banking, and current clinical applications, and it discusses ethical issues and risks.

In: Cord Blood
Editor: Lisandra Vanostrand

ISBN: 978-1-62618-072-7

Chapter 1

Virological Risks and Benefits of Cord Blood Banking

György Berencsi III*, Márta Csire, Katalin Szomor, Erzsébet Barcsay, Katalin Ördög, Mária Takács and János Minárovits

National Center for Epidemiology, Division of Virology, Budapest, Hungary

Abstract

The risks of the reactivation of latently carried maternal viruses during pregnancy and the transfer of primary maternal viral infections to fetus due to the maternal immunomodulation may also affect the safety of the umbilical cord blood banking. Microchymerism, transcytosis, transfer of virus-immunoglobulin complexes and replication of viruses in placental and fetal cells are the mechanisms of the maternal-fetal transfer of viruses.

Very few virus harbouring cells in the cord blood preparations might endanger the health of transplant recipients. Very few cells with latent viruses can be amplified and released during the *in vitro* expansion of the pluripotent umbilical cord blood cell (UCB) populations.

* Postal address: György Berencsi, MD, PhD, Scientific Adviser, Dévai Street 22-24/C, H-1134 BUDAPEST, Hungary. berencsi.gyorgy@gmail.com.

There is a consensus in the literature, that serology only cannot be used for the detection of contaminating viruses. Real time PCR, and or microchips under development seem to be the best, and quickest methodology for this purpose.

It seems to be necessary to broaden the spectrum of viruses to be screened at present. In case the microchip technology will be available, certain interleukins, tumor necrosis factors and interferons might be also included into the preliminary testing. Micro-RNA and or exosome specific molecules might be considered for preliminary testing, since these are indirect markers of virus infections. Viral transactivator proteins TAT, NEF and TAX proteins of HIV1-2 and HTLV 1-4 human retroviruses and HBeAg of hepatitis B virus can pass the placenta and modify cellular function of fetal cells even in the absence of the viruses themselves.

In case the microchip technologies will be routinly introduced, these molecules and also certain lectins (CD161) should be added to the list of viral products, to be tested. The methodology of the UCB control and that of the post-transplantation surveillance has to be completely different.

Contamination with viruses is not always a contraindication to preserve samples. In case appropriate active vaccination for the prevention of the disease or specific chemotherapy are available. This is especially true for enteroviruses, orthomyxoviruses etc. preventable simply by humoral immunity.

Herpesviruses, papillomaviruses, hepatitis B virus, and viruses such as torque teno anellovirus, GB-C/HGV flavivirus, which had not been associated with clinical illnesses.

Transplacental transport of IgG might be useful, but the presence of viruses may reduce the pluripotency of fetal cell clones, certain lymphocyte receptor populations can be eliminated whithout any remarkable signs.

The transfer of anti-idiotypes may induce fetal IgM synthesis in the second half of pregnancy, or eliminate certain clones of germline subgroups of B, NK, T and dendritic cells during the first half of pregnancy.

Maternal virus infections might result fetal modifications (interleukins, exosomes, tumor necrosis factors, interferons) even in the absence of the infection of the fetuses. Maternal-fetal virus transmission was shown to increase from the first trimester untill delivery, the fetal damage, however, is decreasing with time.

The perspectives of the umbilical cord blood transplantation are exponencially improving with the devlopment of molecular and recombination technologies.

Abbreviations

AAV	adeno-associated virus
ADCC	antibody-dependent cellular cytotoxicity
AID	affinity induced deaminase
aGvHD	acute graft versus host disease
AVH	acute viral hepatitis
B-19V	parvovirus B-19 erythrovirus
CCR-1, -3,-5 etc.	chemokine receptors 1, 3, 5
CDR-3	complementary-determining region-3
ciHHV6	chromosomally integrated HHV-6 genome
cMYC	cellular myelocytomatosis protein
CTLs	cytotoxic lymphocytes
EBV	Epstein-Barr virus
EPC	erythroid progenitor cell
epoR	erythropoetin receptor
ER	endoplasmic reticulum
DCs	dendritic cells
FB	fetal blood
FHF	fulminant hepatitis
gB, gH	glycoprotein B and H of HCMV
GvHD	graft versus host disease
HAI	hemagglutination inhibition test
HBcAg	hepatitis B core antigen
HBeAg	hepatitis B e antigen
HBsAg	hepatitis B surface antigen
HBV	hepatitis B virus
HCMV	human cytomegalovirus
HCV	hepatitis C virus
HD	homeodomain
HEV	hepatitis E virus
HGV/GB-C	hepatitis G virus
HHV-6 to -8	human herpesvirus 6 to 8
HIV-1/2	human immundeficiency virus ½
HLA-G	human leukocyt antigen „G" (fetal)
HTLV-1 to 4	human t-cell leukemia/lymphoma virus
ICAM-1	adhesion molecules
IDE	immunodominant epitope
IFN αβγ	interferons α, β and γ

IHS	immune histochemistry
IL2 IL6 etc.	interleukins
iPSC	induced pluripotent stem cell
IVIg	intraveneous immune-globulin
JCV	John Cunningham polyomavirus
KSHV	Kaposi's sarcoma herpesvirus
LACV	La Cross coronavirus
LRTI	lower respiratory tract infections
MAPK	mitogen-activated protein kinase
MAT	myeloablative transplant
MGUS	monoclonal gammopathy of unknown significance
MM	myeloma multiplex
MMF	mycophenolate mofetil
MMR	measles-mumps-rubella vaccine
MPER	membrane-proximal domain
NEF	negative regulatory factor of HIV
NHL	non-Hodgkin lymphoma
NK-cells	natural killer cells
NTDs	neural tube defects
P13K	phosphatidylinositol-3 kinase
PBMC	periferal blood mononuclear cells
PML	progressive multifocal leukoencephalopathy (JCV)
qHPV	qadrivalent human papillomavirus vaccine
RAG-1, -2	recombination-activating genes
RIC	reduced-intensity conditioning
RSV	respiratory syncytial virus
SARS-CoV	severe acute respiratory syndrom coronavirus
STAT5A	signal transducer and activator of transcription 5A
STBM	Syncytiotrophoblast derived microparticles
TAT/TAX	transactivator proteins of retroviruses
TCR	T cell receptor
TNFs	tumor necrosis factors
TRAIL	TNF-related apoptosis-inducing ligand
T_{REG}	regulator T-cell
TTV	torque teno anellovirus
U10, U51, U83 etc.	herpesvirus genes and gene products
UCB	umbilical cord blood
UCBT	unrelated cord blood transplantation
VCAM-1	adhesion molecules

VZV	varicella-zoster virus
WM	Waldenström's macroglobulinemia
WNV	West-Nile virus

Introduction

Umbilical cord blood (UCB) has several advantages over bone marrow (BM) transplantation in a therapeutic setting, particularly the observed lowered incidence of acute graft-versus-host disease (aGvHD) despite the infusion of human leukocyte antigen (HLA) disparate grafts. aGvHD remains a major obstacle to the broader application of allogeneic stem cell therapy and is characterized by donor CD4+ T-cell activation in response to self-antigen presented by class II major histocompatibility complex (MHC) on host antigen-presenting cells (APCs).

IFN-γ expression in cord blood T cells was dependent on the presence of antigen-presenting cells, as addition of IFN-γ during stimulation of purified cord blood T cells did not result in an increase of IFN-γ expression, and depletion of monocytes ablated the rescue of IFN-γ expression (Kadereit et al. 2003). Umbilical cord blood (UCB) graft lymphocyte immune naivety and observed early tolerance induction may contribute to the observed favorable GvHD incidence, despite infusion of HLA mismatch grafts in the unrelated allogeneic setting (Kleen et al. 2005). UCB myeloid and plasmacytoid dendritic cells express only HLA-G mitigating GvHD, in contrast to bone marrow cells and CD34(+) cells which did not produce this molecule (Buzzi et al. 2011).

Before the preparation of cell suspensions for long term storage the *cord blood used to be tested routinly* for the presence of HIV-1/2, hepatitis B virus (HBV), hepatitis C virus (HCV) and in certain cases also for human cytomegalovirus (HCMV). Samples taken in the American continent and in the Far Eastern Countries have to be or should be tested for the presence of the provirus of the human T-cell leukemia/lymphoma virus type 1 (HTLV-1). Time to time West Nile Virus (WNV) or in endemic regions (Italy) Chikungunya or Ross River Virus (Australia) has to be tested, too (Chamberland et al. 2001; Strong and Katz, 2002; Macdonald, 2005; Hema-Québec 2011; Canadian Blood Services, 2011).

This chapter will not discuss *risks of HIV and HCV positive preparations,* since these samples have to be excluded from further utilization. In certain instances even the presence of antiretroviral drugs is tested to exclude undetected transmission of the virus (WHO Recommendations „Preventing HIV Infection in Infants", 2010; Stinson et al. 2012). On the other hand *the presence of hepatitis B virus is no contraindication* of DC preservation and transplantation, since the recipient(s) can be actively immunized and boosted before transplantation. It has been shown recently, that depending on the schedule of immunization of newborns 15 years later 1.9 % to 48.3 % of the students became HBsAg positive.

A significant proportion of complete vaccinees may have lost their immunological memories against HBsAg (Wu et al. 2012). Unfortnately the long term outcome of *intradermal vaccination of newborns with anti-HBs+HBsAg* is not yet known, but it was found to be effective for the first 7 to 15 months of life (Buxmann et al. 2012).

For these persons even *their HBV-containing UCB-graft can be inocuous and life saving.* Nevertheless, the storage conditions of such UCB preparations has to be standardized specifically and realized in separate containers for the prevention of *in vitro* cross-contamination (Hema-Québec, cyt. 2011).

The major *advantages of UCBC transplantations compared with unrelated adult donor* stem cells include more rapid procurement of the graft, the requirement for less-stringent HLA matching, the higher likelihood of finding a match for ethnic minorities, and a decreased incidence of graft-versus-host disease.

Although a major disadvantage of CB is the low stem cell dose, which results in delayed engraftment, there is also delayed immune recovery, particularly in mismatched unrelated cord blood transplantations with the use of antithymocyte globulin. This is attributed to the small numbers of T cells transferred, the absence of memory T cells within the CB grafts, and the apparent hyporesponsiveness of CB antigen-presenting cells. Consequently, CB recipients are susceptible to an array of viral and other infections that are the leading cause of death in these patients (Szabolcs and Niedzwiecki, 2007; Walker et al. 2007).

The unique features of immune reconstitution following *unrelated cord blood transplantation (UCBT)* that lead to heightened risk of infection-related mortality in the early post-UCBT period. There is no evidence that innate immunity is uniquely compromised after UCBT, but the development of antigen-specific cellular immunity is affected by numerical and qualitative deficits, primarily within the first 100 days (Reviewed by Szabolcs and Cairo, 2010).

The Mechanisms of Maternal-Fetal Infections with Human Viruses

The *vertical transmission* of chromosomally integrated human herpesvirus 6 (ciHHV-6) into the telomeres of chromosomes follows the Mendelian rules of inheritance (Tanaka-Taya et al. 2004; de Pagter et al. 2010; Hall et al. 2010; Arbuckle et al. 2010, 2012). In mesenchymal stromal stem cell preparations *in vitro* expanded for transplantation, however, no unintegrated HHV-6 virus was detected (Pessina et al. 2009). *Adeno-associated viruses (AAV)* used to be carried covalently integrated into chromosome 19 (Hüser and Heilbronn, 2003). The persons borne after chromosomal transmission of viruses possess no virus-specific serological markers, unless reactivation occurs during fetal life or after birth or organ transplantation (Kobayashi et al. 2011).

It has been proven, that the clinical disease caused by both HHV-6 and 7 is *Pityriasis rosea* (Watanabe et al. 2002). HHV-6, but not HHV-7 DNA could be detected in pregnants suffering from *Pityriasis rosea* and aborted within the first 15 weeks of pregnancy. Adenovirus, EBV and HCMV DNA and enterovirus RNA in fetal tissues has been tested first in pathological pregnancies (Wenstrom et al. 1998; Van den Veyver et al. 1998). Transplacental transmission was confirmed in the case of HHV-6, too (Broccolo et al. 2005; Drago et al. 2008).

Midtrimester amniotic fluid was tested for adenovirus, cytomegalovirus, respiratory syncytial virus, enterovirus, Epstein-Barr virus, and parvovirus B19 using multiplex PCR . Amniotic fluid viral PCR testing was suggested for fetuses with intrauterine growth restriction, nonimmune hydrops fetalis, hand/foot anomalies, or neural tube defects (NTDs) after aneuploidy had been excluded. PCR was found to be positive in 6.5 % of the tested pregnants. Adenovirus was most frequently identified (37/44), followed by CMV (5/44), EBV (2/44), enterovirus (2/44) and RSV (1/44) in the midtrimester amniotic fluid of sonographically normal fetus. The prevalence followed a seasonal pattern with the exception of adenoviruses (Petrikovsky et al. 2003; Baschat et al. 2003a and b; Reddy et al. 2005; Adams et al. 2012).

Later at birth following complication-free pregnancy the amniotic fluid of 35 of 106 healthy newborns was found to be positive for EBV, HCMV, HHV-6, -7, -8 and human papillomaviruses (HpaV) DNA (Table 1) indicating the inocuity of the viruses, but its increasing capability to pass the placental barriere (Younes et al. 2007). The situation is probably different following organ transplantation and immunosuppression, since in 9 of 22 liver transplant recipients HHV-7 reactivation occurred within 90 days after the surgical operation and the symptomatology was found to be similar to HCMV reactivation (Peigo et al. 2005). It has been shown, that *human parvovirus B-19 (B-19V)* invades the amniotic cavity in the midtrimester of pregnancy (Gervasi et al. 2012).

Episomal viral genomes or virions (papilloma- or polyomavirus) were found to be present in the sperm cells or adsorbed to spermatozoa and transferred into the zygote (Brackett et al. 1971; Foresta et al. 2010, 2011a and b, Syrjänen, 2010).

The maternofetal transplacental transmission was shown to occur in connection with *microchymerism* reviewed recently (Berencsi and Barcsay, 2012). Lymphotropic herpesviruses and human retroviruses can be transfered by latently infected maternal B and T lymphocytes into the fetus without any clinical symptoms or any sign of virus replication. Hepatitis C virus infection of 1-3 % of the newborns of RNA-negative women might occur transplacentally because of maternal-fetal microchimerism (Hurtado et al. 2010).

Transplacental Transmission of Viruses and Virus-Coded Products

Transplacental transmission occurs most frequently through the infection of decidual cells or direct polarized transfer (transcytosis) of the viruses through the syncytiotrophoblast (reviewed by Berencsi and Csire, 2012; Csire M, Mikala, 2012). Type B enteroviruses (King et al. 2000), flaviviruses (West-Nile virus), Japanese encephalitis virus (JEV) and Ross River virus (Chaturvedi et al. 1980, Aaskov et al. 1981; CDC-report, 2002) were found to be transmitted transplacentally. The overall rate of mother-to-child transmission of hepatitis C virus (2-6%) is strikingly low (Hurtado et al. 2010). Torque teno anellovirus (TTV) DNA could be detected in amniotic fluid and/or cord blood (Toyoda et al. 1999; Iso et al. 2001; Matsubara et al. 2001). Some of the health care workers were shown to carry TTV virus for 10 years without any clinical symptoms (Dencs et al. 2009). It is not surprizing, that about 50 % of the amniotic fluids of healthy newborns was found to be PCR positive (Csire M and Dencs A, unpublished, 2009).

Direct detection of the viral DNA in the amniotic fluid Table 1. support the existance of transplacental transmission of herpesviruses (EBV, HCMV, HHV-6, HHV-7, Kaposi sarcoma herpesvirus, papillomaviruses and torque teno virus) in healthy pregnancies (Younes et al. 2007; Vamvakas, 2010;

Trottier et al. 2012). Recently papillomaviruses have been identified in 8.3 % of adult blood samples, suggesting, that the PBMC-adsorbed papillomaviruses might be also a source of transplacental transmission since papillomaviruses could be detected in the cells of the placenta and cord blood (Sarkola et al. 2008; Chen et al. 2009). Adeno-associated defective virus (AAV) has been also detected in fetal tissues (Burguete et al. 1999).

Table 1. Detection of human herpes- and papillomaviruses in the amniotic fluid (Younes et al. 2007)

Virus detected in	Amniotic fluid (106)	Maternal blood (106)
Epstein-Barr virus	4	1
Human Cytomegalov.	9	1
Human Herpesv. -6	1	3
Human Herpesv. -7	8	1
Human Herpesv. -8	5	7
Human papilloma virus	8	Sarkola et al. 2008; Chen et al. 2009
Total	35	13

Hepatitis B virus (HBV) translocates across a trophoblastic barrier (Bhat and Anderson, 2007; Yogeswaran and Fung. 2011; Bhat P, 2012). Outcome of perinatal hepatitis B virus exposure was dependent on maternal virus load (Burk et al. 1994). In mothers with high viral load, vertical infection *in utero* could be prevented by lamivudine, telbivudine or tenofovir treatment (Pol et al. 2011).The chronic virus carrier state of the newborn could be prevented by combined active and passive immunisation on the 1st day of life (Delage and Carter 1992; Kékesi et al. 1993; Romano et al. 2011). The nationwide introduction of serological screening and activ-passive immunization reduced the transplacental and perinatal transmission of HBV below 1 % in the newborns (Straub 1996). The transplacental HBV-transmission was shown not to be the reason for vaccination failure, since from 16 DNS-positive babies only one had HBV DNA in the prenatal amniotic fluid and cord blood samples (Zhu et al. 2010). A systemic review have been prepared on the basis of eight controlled studies recently by Shi and coworkers. It has been concluded, that hepatitis B virus will not be transfered to the newborns in connection with breast feeding, when the newborns have been vaccinated actively and passively upon birth (Shi et al. 2011; Zheng et al. 2011).

Maternal HBeAg was shown to be transmitted into the fetal circulation, too. In the presence of maternal HBeAg the immune response of the newborns was severly impaired (Tseng et al. 2011). The authors suggested earlier that the transplacental maternal HBeAg probably induces a specific unresponsiveness of helper T cells to HBcAg and HBeAg in the neonates born to HBeAg-positive carrier mothers. This specific helper T cell tolerance could be maintained throughout the early replicative phase of carrier state but might break someday with the appearance of raised ALT level (Hsu et al. 1992). This idea can now be completed with the hypotetic possibility of the maternal-fetal transfer of T_{REG} –cells by microchymerism. The existance of specific breakage has been proven later and the possible role of idiotype/anti-idiotype network has been suggested as the possible mechanism of it (Ördög et al. 2003; Reviewed by Berencsi and Ördög, 2012; Table 2).

The observed inhibitory effect of maternal HBeAg to the seroconversion of the offspring (Tseng et al. 2011) might have a complex mechanism involving maternal-fetal microchymerism (T_{REG}-cells), anti-idiotypes (antigenic mimicry), development of fetal immunotolerance and HLA and IL-genotypes of the newborn as suggested earlier (Wu et al. 2006; Wu et al. 2011). Recently it has been suggested, that a significant proportion of adolescents vaccinated at birth with active HBV vaccine and hepatitis B immunoglobulin have lost their specific immunological memory and responded poorly to the revaccination at 15 years of age (Wang and Lin, 2007; Wu et al. 2012).

The authors of this chapter suggest, that the fetal contact with the maternal-fetal transfer of HBeAg and HBsAg might be responsible for the modulation of the immune response.

Fetal ascites can be caused by maternal hepatitis virus infections including *hepatitis E virus (HEV)*. Cord blood was found to be positive for HEV-specific IgM, but no virus could be detected any more at birth (Pradhan et al. 2012). The HEV viral load was significantly higher in pregnants suffering from fulminant hepatitis (FHF) than in acute viral hepatitis (AVH) ($p<0.001$) and in cases with fetal mortality in AVH. The risk of fetal mortality in AVH was two times and maternal and fetal mortalities in FHF were 4-fold higher in the case of carriers of progesterone receptor gene mutations. The expression of progesteron receptor and that of progesteron induced blocking factor was found to be lower in AVH and even lower in FHF compared to healthy controls. (Bose et al. 2011).

Latent HBV transmission has been observed undetectable using only serological methods (Kwon et al. 2008). The mechanism of mother to infant transmission of lymphotropic „*hepatitis G virus (GB-C/HGV)* has not been examined in detail, but vertical transmission could be reduced, but not eliminated after caesarean section (Ohto et al. 2000).

Maternal-fetal transmission of *chikungunya virus* has been documented during the recent epidemics (Lenglet et al. 2006; Touret et al. 2006; Gerardin et al. 2008). Maternofetal transmission of *human coronaviruses* has been suggested in a pilot study (Gagneur et al. 2008).

In vitro SARS Coronavirus induced the expression of CCR-1, CCR-3, and CCR-5 chemokine receptors. There was also strong induction of TNF-related apoptosis-inducing ligand (TRAIL), but not Fas ligand gene expression in SARS-CoV infected dendritic cells (DCs). Interestingly, the expressions of most genes studied were higher in UCB DCs than in adult DCs (Law et al. 2009).

Yellow fever vaccine was found to be transmitted by breast milk, and the infection caused meningoencephalitis (Traiber et al. 2011). The vaccination against yellow fever, however, was not recommended during pregnancy.

Quadrivalent HPV (qHPV) vaccine-induced antibodies cross the placenta and could potentially provide some benefit against vaccine-type HPaV infection and related diseases such as recurrent respiratory papillomatosis (Matys et al. 2012).

One has to realize, that even *arteficial nanoparticles* have been shown to penetrate in *ex vivo* experiments trophoblast cells through differentiated channels (Kertschanska et al. 1997).

Polarized passage through the syncytiotrophoblast can occur in the form of *virus-IgG complexes* i.e. human cytomegalovirus (HCMV) utilizing the mechanism of maternal-fetal IgG transport (Maidji et al. 2006, 2007, 2010; Pereira et al. 2007). Only individual virus particles and non-neutralizing IgG complexes were found to be transmitted this way. Immunglobulin treatment with HCMV-sepcific preparations were found to mitigate pathologic and clinical consequences, but the infection of fetus could not be prevented (Maidji et al. 2010). The transplacental transmission of HCMV is frequent in the 3rd trimester of pregnancy, but without clinical consequences in the wast majority of pregnants (Enders et al. 2011).

Maternal *preconceptional HCMV seropositivity cannot prevent fetal infection.* Virus reactivation occurs regularly due to the immunomodulation of the pregnants. Evidence has been presented, that subsequent pregnancies can be affected by the same reactivated HCMV strain (Nagamori et al. 2010). Superinfection of the pregnant with different HCMV subtypes may occur, too (Boppana et al. 2001; Fowler et al. 2003; Kenneson and Cannon 2007). The possibility of an infection occurring in the first trimester with the subsequent loss of IgM cannot be excluded. The incidence of primary infection among pregnant women ranges from 0.5% and 4% (Peckham 1991). In connection with organ transplantation it has been observed, that the adverse events were more frequent in the donor+/recipient+ pairs, than in the case of donor+/recipient- pairs. The explanation of this phenomenon is simple, but its laboratory examination is difficult. The main neutralization epitopes of HCMV are located on the gB and gH glycoproteins. The gH protein was shown to be responsible for the fusion of the viral envelop and the membrane of the recipient cell. Strain specific heterogeneity was found to be present on the epitopes located at the first 37 amino acids of gH. The gB protein possesses both conserved (68 to 77 aa and 560 to 640 aa) and variable strain specific epitopes (50 to 54 aa) reviewed recently by Ishibashi et al. (2007, 2011). The antibody response specific to HCMV subtypes is further modified by the HLA haplotype of the individuals. Recently a real-time PCR technique has been also developed for the differentiation of the subtypes of the gH gene (Ikuta et al. 2012).

The HCMV glycoprotein US10 transmembrane protein inserted into the endoplasmic reticulum (ER) membrane selectively targets HLA-G for degradation, but the expression of MHC class-I was not influenced by it (Park et al. 2010).

Maternal-fetal *perinatal virus* infections is not any more the subject of the present review, since its definition is the fetal infection with reactivated viruses of the genital tract of the pregnant during delivery (Czeglédy et al. 1989; Cason et al. 1998; El-Sageyer et al. 1998; Rice et al. 1999, 2000; Czeglédy 2001; Koskimaa et al. 2012; Syrjänen, 2010; Yoshida et al. 2011).

In connection with the recently discovered *KI, WU, and Merkel cell polyomaviruses* no evidence of mother-to-fetus transmission have been detected (Sadeghi et al. 2010).

The main advantage of immune histochemistry (IHS) is that it allowed confirmation of BKV infection diagnosis in urine samples. Immunohistochemistry staining (IHS) detected more BKV-infected cells in samples with few positive urothelial cells, which would have gone undetected if only Papanicolaou staining had been used as the BKV screening method. Urine samples testing for BKV by both techniques will improve diagnosis in asymptomatic patients, allowing early therapeutic intervention and a better clinical outcome (Yuste et al. 2008).

Reactivation of the John Cunningham virus (JCV) under conditions of cellular immuno-compromise in patients with acquired immunodeficiency syndrome (AIDS) or organ transplant recipients the progressive multifocal leuko-encephalopathy (PML) related to resonance imaging demonstrated marked signal abnormality in deficits rapidly increased JCV encephalitis must be early suspected (El-Cheikh et al. 2012).

Table 2. Detection of viruses in the amniotic fluid or cord blood of healthy fetuses

Virus	Circumstances	References		
None	1st trimester	McLean et al. 1995		
AAV	At delivery	Burguete et al. 1999		
EBV	2nd-3rd trimester	de-Thé, 1977	Younes et al. 2007	Trottier et al. 2012
HBV	transcytosis	Bhat and Armstrong, 2009	Kwon et al. 2008	
HCV	sarcoma-chymerism			
HGV/GB-C	long term, symptomeless	Ohto et al. 2000		
HHV-6	Second trimester	Younes et al. 2007	Gervain et al. 2012	Arbuckle et al. 2010, 2012
HHV-7	At delivery	Younes et al. 2007	Peigo et al. 2009	
HHV-8	At delivery	Younes et al. 2007	Vamvakas, 2010	
HCMV	2dn-3rd trimester	Gervasi et al. 2012	Younes et al. 2007	Kourí et al. 2010
HParvovirus	2nd trimester	Gervasi et al. 2012	Weiffenbach J et al. 2012	
HPapillomavirus	At delivery	Burguette et al. 1999	Younes et al. 2007	
HTLV-1 to 4	2nd-3rd trimester			
Adenovirus		Van de Veyver et al. 1998	Wenstrom et al. 1998	Reddy et al. 2005
Enterovirus	transcytosis, delivery	Petrikovsky et al. 2003	Baschat et al. 2000, 2003	El-Sageyer et al. 1998
RSV		Baschat et al. 2000, 2003		
TTV	long term symptomless	Matsubara et al. 2001	Iso et al. 2001	Dencs et al. 2009

HTLV-1 is transmitted mainly through prolonged breastfeeding, and such infection represents a major risk for the development of adult T-cell leukemia/lymphoma.

Free infectious HTLV-1 virions, however, could cross the epithelial barrier via a transcytosis mechanism. Such virions were able to infect productively human dendritic cells located beneath the epithelial barrier (Martin-Latil et al. 2012).

Evidence has been presented in tropical spastic paraparesis patients that antibody mimicry and activation of cytotoxic T cells by the TAX protein are participating in the pathogenesis of HTLV-1 associated autoimmune myelopathy (Domínguez et al. 2008; Nakamura, 2009).

It has been also clarified as early as in 1969, that the *attenuated rubella vaccine virus can pass the placenta,* can be isolated from the fetal tissues, but no rubella syndrome was ever caused by the MMR vaccine virus (Vaheri et al. 1969, 1972; Bozzo et al. 2011). Evidence has been provided against the association of autism with either MMR or a single measles vaccine (Mrozek-Budzyn et al. 2010). These vaccinations, however, are not considered as an indication for termination of the pregnancy (Sur et al. 2003; Nasiri et al. 2009).

The absence of vertical hantavirus transmission was demonstrated recently in pregnant women with onset of hantavirus disease between gestation weeks 14 and 28 (Hofmann et al. 2012). It has been proven, however, that the flue epidemics are responsible for fetal impairments simply because of the elevation of the body temperature of the pregnants (Acs et al. 2005).

Time Course of Maternal-Fetal Virus Infections

In the first trimester of pregnancy only very few viruses can infect the fetus. In the majority of cases, the virus infection is lethal for the fetus, but the maternal symptoms were found to be usually absent or very mild (i.e. rash or polyarthralgy between the 5th to 17th week of pregnancy). The ultrasonographic symptoms of fetuses were documented on the 17th to 23rd week of pregnancy (hyperechogenic bowel, ascites or cerebral ventriculomegaly). Neither the specific IgM, nor the DNA testing of the maternal sera revealed all maternofetal *parvovirus B-19* infections (Enders et al. 2007; de Jong et al. 2011; Bonvicini et al. 2011). In addition to this, the *epidemiological cycles* of the viruses in the population (5-7 years according to I. Mezey, personal communication) play an important role. In Norway only

0.7 % of stillbirth was found to be caused by parvovirus B-19 (erythrovirus) using serological approach (Sarfraz et al. 2009).

Infection by B19V is restricted exclusively to human erythroid progenitor cells (EPCs) both in the maternal bone marrow and in the fetal organism where the EPCs are replicating in the fetal liver (Takahashi et al. 1990). A model of ''rolling hairpin''- dependent DNA replication of B19V has been proposed (Cotmore SF and Tattersall P, 2005). Epo and the Epo receptor (EpoR) serves as a molecular switch for B19V DNA replication in cells which have internalized the virus (Chen et al. 2010a). Janus kinase 2 activates a kinase cascade with three major branches, starting at the signal transducer and activator of transcription 5A (STAT5A), mitogen-activated protein kinase (ERK/MAPK) kinase (MEK) and phosphatidylinositol-3kinase (PI3K). *Ex vivo* expanded CD36+ EPCs cultured in the context of hypoxia (1% oxygen) support sustained productive B19V infection, efficiently amplifying the numbers of infectious virions within the cell by enhancing the level of viral DNA replication. STAT5A was found to be critical in promoting hypoxia-facilitated B19V infection in CD36+ EPCs during erythropoiesis, whereas MEK kinase negatively regulated B19V infection. In addition to these the virus-coded nonstructural 11K protein was found to be responsible for the apoptosis of the infected reticulocytes (Chen et al 2010a and b, 2011). The risk of invasive diagnostic procedures have been summarized recently by Lopéz and Coll (2010).

The B-lymphocyte premalignancies and malignancies of plasma cell origin emphasize the role of latently harboured HHV-8 Kaposi's sarcoma herpesvirus (Table 3) in comparison to the non-Hodgkin lymphoma patients (Csire et al. 2007).

It is not surprising, that without molecular technology HHV-8 cannot be detected only in 13 % of the myeloma multiplex patients (Sadeghian et al. 2008). Developing B cells normally exhibit a short life span and a high rate of turnover in which gammaherpesviruses may gain access to the mature B cell compartment by recurrent seeding of developing B cells (Coleman et al. 2010). The results presented in Table 3 suggest, that the serology cannot be used for the detection of KSHV (HHV-8) carier state of the patients or recipients.

Of 28 pediatric heart and heart-lung transplant recipients; of mean age 11.5 +/- 2.5 years all patients were seronegative pretransplantation. Ten seroconversions occurred within the third year after transplantation (Concato et al. 2008).

Table 3. Frequency of EBV, HCMV, HHV-6 and HHV-8 PCR-positivity of PBMC in patients with multiple myeloma (MM), monoclonal gammopathy of unknown significance (MGUS) and Waldenström's macroglobulinemia (WM) in comparison to the non-Hodgkin lymphoma controls (Csire et al. 2007)

Virus	EBV	HCMV	HHV-6	HHV-8
MM+MGUS+WM	40/95 (42.1 %)	19/95 (20.0 %)	17/95 (17.9 %)	40/95 (42.1 %)
Non-Hodgkin-L	23/44 (52.3 %)	4/44 (9.1 %)	8/44 (18.2 %)	1/44 (2.3 %)
P value	non significant	non significant	non significant	P < 0.0004

On the basis of the listed results the authors of this chapter suggest, that the donors have been transplacentally infected with HHV-8 (KSHV) and the immunotolerant state prevented the serological detection of the carrier state. In addition to these Kaposi's sarcoma herpesvirus DNA could be detected in the PBMC preparations of patients suffering from B-cell abnormalities as shown in Table 3. The proportion of EBV, HCMV and HHV-6 PCR positivity was found to be comparable in the patients and in the PBMCs of patients suffering from Non-Hodkin Lymphoma (NHL) controls in contrast to HHV-8, which could be detected in 42.1 % of PBMC of pateints suffering from *myeloma multiplex*(MM), monoclonal gammopathy of unknown significance (MGUS) and Waldenström's macroglobulinemia (WM), but only 1 of 44 NHL patients carried the HHV-8 virus in PBMCs. In contrast to EBV, HCMV and HHV-6 seropositivity of patients, only 3 of the the HHV-8-carriers were found to be seropositive (Csire et al. 2007).

Recently the substantial alteration of NK cell receptor repertoire in healthy HHV8 carriers, with reduced expression of NKp30, NKp46 and CD161 (lectin) receptors. In addition, down-modulation of the activating NKG2D receptor, associated with impaired NK-cell lytic capacity have been published probably facilitating tumor development (Dupuy et al. 2012).

Virus-Specific IgM and Germline Antibodies in the Cord Blood

Cord blood contains germline antibodies or antibodies with very low level of somatic hypermutations. In the second half of the pregnancy, however, measurable amounts of virus-specific IgM populations can be produced, which can be detected by conventional serological techniques. Cord blood and infant heel-stick blood samples were positive for WNV-specific IgM and neutralizing antibodies (CDC-report, 2002). HIV-1 could have evolved to elude strong binding to minimally somatically-diversified human antibodies as an escape mechanism from adaptive immune responses in contrast to SARS-CoV or Hendra virus-specific antibodies (Xiao et al. 2009; Chen et al. 2012). One can hypothesize, that the glycoprotein epitopes of the surface proteins of HIV-1 have suffered similar adaptation at the level of the germline antibodies, similar to the T-cell epitopes of the internal proteins of influenza A virus subtypes. About 30 amino-acid T-cell epitopes have been found in the internal proteins of influenza A/H1N1/2009 to those of human enzymes recently (Heiny et al. 2007; Tan et al. 2010). The probability of a positive B19V-IgG or B19V-IgM finding in fetal blood increased with gestational age (Weiffenbach et al. 2012). Dengue virus specific IgM was found in the cord blood of 1 of 64 IgM+ pregnants (Tan et al. 2008). Fortunately the newborn had no clinical signs of infection. Human cytomegalovirus infection of the fetus cannot be diagnosed on the basis of neither maternal, nor fetal IgM. The only safe procedure was found to be the DNA detection in the amniotic fluid or the direct DNA PCR of the cord blood (Albano et al. 2006; Theiler et al. 2006; Al-Hareth et al. 2009; Adler, 2011; Yoshida et al. 2012).

Seven (2.7%) were considered to have a *varicella zoster virus (VZV)* fetal infection. (Trlifajova et al. 1986; Sanches et al. 2011). An overall prevalence for infectious disease markers of 6%; IgM anti-HCMV was the most prevalent, representing 5% of total units in Mexico (Jaime-Pérez et al. 2012). In a Chinese Blood Bank in Guangzhou only 0.5 % HCMV-specific IgM positivity has been found (Wu et al. 2006). In other publications no HCMV-specific IgM could be found, therefore one has to suppose the different sensitivities and specificities of the methodology used.

Many cytokine responses varied by season of birth, including 2–3 fold fluctuations with specific IFN-α and IFN-γ responses. Birthweight was inversely associated with *post partum* IFN-γ responses to *respiratory syncytium virus (RSV),* but positively associated with IL-8 responses to a variety of innate stimuli. Maternal autoimmune diseases caused reduced cytokine levels in umbilical cord blood (Setiady et al. 2003; Gold et al. 2009).

Congenital *La Cross Bunyavirus (LACV)* infection of the fetus was suggested through identification of IgM antibodies in umbilical cord serum, although the newborn was asymptomatic and development was normal. Although unlikely to cross the placental barrier, LACV IgM antibodies detected in cord serum might have been attributable to transplacental leakage induced by uterine contractions that disrupt placental barriers during labor, which has been documented for anti-Toxoplasma IgM antibodies (Pinon et al. 2001; CDC-MMWR, 2009).

Differences in the Virus-Specific IgG Present in the Cord Blood

IgG antibodies specific to different epitopes and domains on gp41 protein of HIV-1 subtype C exist at various titers were found to neutralize HIV *in vitro* and inhibit transcytosis. It could be found in HIV-uninfected babies born to HIV-infected mothers. The antibody titres of non-infected cord bloods were significantly lower against the membrane-proximal (MPER) domain of gp41 and specific to its disulfide loop immunodominant epitope (IDE) and were probaly associated with HIV-1/C exposure without infection (Diomede et al. 2012). In addition to these, the maternal HIV-1/2 infection is able to facilitate transmission of many other viruses into the HIV-1/2 negative fetuses (Miller et al. 2012).

The lack of B19V-IgG in fetuses with parvovirus B19V-derived anemia or hydrops is most likely due to a limited maternal-fetal transfer of IgG and a poor fetal antibody response. Fetal B19V infection is poorly controlled in the absence of specific antibodies (Weiffenbach et al. 2012). Parvovirus B19 infection in pregnancy have been reviewed recently by De Jong et al. (2011).

The data provide an explanation, why intraveneous treatment of the pregnants with gamma globulin (Selbing et al. 1995; Rugolotto et al. 1999) or IgG-enriched hyperimmune gamma globulin preparations can improve the clinical status of the fetuses suffering from severe B19V anemia (Matsuda et al. 2005). It was proven, that the gamma globulin inoculated intraamnially was detected in the cord blood upon birth. Even IgG2 and IgG4 has been actively transported into the fetal circulation (Yoshida et al. 2011).

In comparison to maternal plasma, IgG1 and high avidity neutralizing HCMV-specific antibodies were found to be selectively enriched in umbilical cord blood samples (Nozawa et al. 2009). The main problem of the screenenig programmes for the prevention of maternal fetal HCMV transmission is, that the seropositive pregnants are screened only at the beginning of pregnancy. The pregnants seronegative for both specific IgG and IgM are only retested in the second and third trimesters.

This regime could identify 27 pregnants of 83 pregnants suffering from primary infection (Kourí et al. 2010). This serological approach cannot detect 1.) HCMV reactivations ; 2.) Superinfections with new HCMV subtypes (Stagno et al. 1977; Fowler et al. 1982, 2003); 3.) Reactivated maternal HCMV transcytosed through the placenta in the form of IgG-HCMV complexes (Maidji et al. 2006, 2007, 2010; Pereira et al. 2007), and 4.) Transplacental transfer of microchymeric cells latently harbouring circular HCMV DNA (Reviewed by Younes et al. 2009; Berencsi and Barcsay, 2011).

On the basis of the amniotic fluid tests (Younes et al. 2007) at the very end of the healthy pregnancies 8.49 % of the amniotic fluids contained HCMV DNA. The samples were taken before the arteficial rupture of the membranes using vacutainers, therefore the external contamination has been excluded. On the basis of these findings one can conclude, that from 83 seronegative pregnants 27 (32,5 %) has suffered primary HCMV infections in Cuba. From the total of 1131 pregnant women had probably HCMV DNA in the amniotic fluid before delivery, i.e. 69 seropositive pregnants had HCMV reactivation or superinfection during pregnancy (Kourí et al. 2010).

A similar screening regime has been used in an urban district of Northern-Italy (de Paschale et al. 2009). They have included the screening of HCMV-specific IgG avidity, too. They have tested 2817 pregnants in the 1st trimester. In 67 % (1899) of them seropositivity could be detected. The number of pregnants tested in the 2nd and 3rd trimester was lower than the initial cohort. The number of IgM seroconverters was found to be 29 of 893 (3.2 %). The avidity tests enabled the identification of 13 reactivations or primary infections. According to the amniotic fluid data of Younes et al. (2007) 161 unrecognized reactivations could be predicted.

In Catalonia, Spain umbilical cord blood samples has been tested for the presence of protective levels of measles antibodies using IgG-specific ELISA and it was found to be above 95 % (Plans et al. 2010).

Virus-Specific Cytotoxic T-Cells in the Cord Blood

Virus-specific T cells could not be generated from cord blood, probably due to the absence of virus-specific memory T cells. This problem has been solved by introducing recombinant adenoviruses expressing Epsein-Barr virus or cytomegalovirus antigens (Hanley et al. 2012).

Abnormal expression of the *Hoxb2* and *Hoxb4* genes induced by HCMV may play important roles in abnormal hematopoietic damage (Liu et al. 2011). A number of variables were studied to identify other *risk factors for HCMV reactivation* in the transplant recipients. This included median age, male sex, diagnosis, sibling versus matched unrelated donor, use of bone marrow versus PBSC or cord blood as graft source, reduced-intensity conditioning (RIC) versus conventional myeloablative transplant (MAT), type of GvHD prophylaxis (mycophenolate mofetil versus non-MMF regimens), use of anti-thymocyte globulin and alemtuzumab during conditioning, HCMV serostatus pre-transplant, and presence of acute GvHD. On univariate analysis the significant risk factors identified included high-risk CMV serostatus (P<0.001), use of alemtuzumab during conditioning (P= 0.03), and the presence of acute GvHD (P< 0.0001). The use of RIC regimen was associated with a higher incidence of HCMV reactivation (45.7%) versus 35.2% with MAT, though the difference was not statistically signifcant (George et al. 2010).

"Vitamin D" deficiency in healthy neonates is associated with increased risk of respiratory syncytial virus (RSV) associated lower respiratory tract infections (LRTI) after birth in the first year of life (Belderbos et al. 2011). Intensified routine vitamin D supplementation during pregnancy may be a useful strategy to prevent RSV LRTI during infancy (Hollis and Pittard, 1984; Adorini et al. 2003; Roth et al. 2008). 1,25-dihydroxyvitamin D3 (1,25-vitD) reprograms *dendritic cells (DC) to become tolerogenic.* The vitamin D and its receptor induced 1,25-vitD sensitive genes in early phases of differentiation if the precursor is present. Exogenous or endogenously generated 1,25-vitD regulated a large set of its targets, the chemokine CCL22, the inhibitory receptors CD300LF and CYP24A1 leading to the tolerogenic state of monocyte derived dendritic cells (DCs) (Széles et al. 2009). Peripheral blood DC subsets, plasmacytoid DCs and CD11c1 myeloid DCs in the response against HCMV. These DCs, rather than being paralyzed by HCMV, are largely resistant to infection, mount vigorous first-line defense and induce T-cell responses to the virus providing the highly efficient control of viral infection and reactivation in immunocompetent hosts in spite of multi-layered viral evasion mechanisms (Rölle and Olweus, 2009).

Expression of *CD161 lectin (NKRP1A)* on circulating virus-specific T cells in patients with hepatitis B and C was observed, and the levels were higher on the tissue-infiltrating populations of such cells. Such expression was not found on T cells specific for most other viruses tested, including HIV, HCMV, and EBV. CD161 expression might define a subset of CD8+T-cells with a distinct differentiation program, leading to a novel phenotype, homing, and function. This T cell lineage that is present already in cord blood and represents as many as one in six circulating CD8+T-cells in healthy humans (Lanier et al. 1994; Northfield et al. 2008; Billerbeck et al. 2010).

Leptin levels in cord blood of healthy neonates was found to be associated with IFN-γ production by cord blood T-cells (Mouzaki et al. 2012).

Oligoclonality characterizes differentiated (CD27-CD28-) γδT cells from HCMV-infected newborns expressing highly the transcription factor T-bet and producing high levels of IFN-γ. γδT cells are unconventional T cells that can react rapidly upon activation and show major histocompatibility complex–

unrestricted activity. Upon HCMV infection *in utero*, fetal γδT cells expand and become differentiated. Their clones are carrying the CDR3γ8 excess sequence of germline encoded complementary-determining region-3 (CDR3) δ1–CALGELGDDKLIF/CDR3γ-8–CATWDTTGWFKIF of 11 excess amino acids. Differentiated γδT cells and public Vγ8Vδ1-TCReceptors were detected as early as after 21 weeks of gestation. The authors suggest that functional fetal that development of this T cell subsets could participate in antiviral defense in early life (Vermijlen et al. 2010).

IgG-opsonized HCMV virions induced IFNγ production of CD16(+)γδ T cells, but did not mediate ADCC against HCMV-infected cells. This CD16-induced IFNγ production was greatly enhanced by IL12 and IFNα, 2 cytokines produced during HCMV infection, and conferred to γδ T cells the ability to inhibit HCMV multiplication in vitro (Couzi et al. 2012).

All this molecular and cellular modifications are important for the postnatal life of the newborn, and for the therapeutical effect of cord blood cell preparations.

Influence of Viruses to the Cord Blood Cell Populations

Coronavirus, cytomegalovirus, herpes simplex virus, influenza virus, morbillivirus blocked Th2 (IL-13) production of cord blood CD4(+) cells. Enveloped viruses were able to impaire Th2 responses in human cord T cells, but IFN-α secretion (innate Th1 response) in cord blood cells was only induced by *S. aureus* and influenza virus (Svennsson et al 2012).

Syncytiotrophoblast derived microparticles (STBMs). STBMs interact with both immune and endothelial cells and may contribute to the systemic inflammation of both normal and pre-eclamptic pregnancies. However inhibitory activity has also been ascribed to trophoblast derived exosomes. *In vitro*, they down-regulate T cell activity, a T cell change that has been repeatedly observed, *ex vivo*, during normal pregnancy (Denzer et al. 2000; Redman and Sargent, 2008). After normal delivery a slight elevation of microparticles has been observed by (Schweintzger et al. 2011). *Syncytin-1 of microsomal membranes* coded for by human endogeneous retrovirus W (HERV-W) was found to be responsible for the *activation of T-cells and PBMCs*. Production of chemokines and interleukins indicated the modulation of the basal peripheral immune cell activation and induction of responsiveness to LPS during normal pregnancy by placental microvesicles carrying syncytin-1 (Holder et al. 2012a and b). Exosomes containing *glycoprotein 350 released by EBV-transformed B cells* selectively target B cells through CD21 and block EBV infection *in vitro* (Vallhov et al. 2011). Rituximab, a monoclonal antibody specific to CD20 was shown to reduce EBV DNAemia in the treated pregnants and reduce the number of maternal-fetal microchimerism (Coppoletta et al. 2010). The recipients EBV-reactivation triggered GvHD could be significantly reduced by the transfusion of maternal EBV-positive lymphocytes in case the previous fetomaternal infection through microchymerism could be detected (Wang et al. 2010).

EBV-associated posttransplantation lymphoma after cord blood-transplantation could be treated successfully with monocyte/natural killer cell–depleted mononuclear cells stimulated *in vitro* at a 20:1 ratio with irradiated autologous EBV-transformed B-cell lines (EBV-BLCLs). After 11 days, T cells were restimulated weekly with irradiated EBV-BLCLs at a 4:1 ratio with interleukin-2. After Rituximab therapy and at least 28 days, T cells were tested for EBV-specificity and CTLs of the closest HLA-match to the UCB donor (and hence the lymphoma) that were restricted by 1 or more of that donor's HLA-alleles were selected for administration (Barker et al. 2010).

Myelosuppression caused by HCMV infection has been detected (Simmons et al. 1990; Randolph-Habecker at al. 2002). Certain HCMV strains induce high amounts of IL-8, which in turn enhances HCMV replication in the placenta, while others can replicate if the IL-8 is provided by a co-infecting agent. The number of nuclei of the syncytiotrophoblast positive for HCMV immediate early antigen (IE) was found to be proportional to the concentration of IL8 in the medium (Kovács et al. 2007). The fetal pathogenicity of the HCMV might be the consequence of the fact, that the expression of 88 genes of *fetal dendritic cells (DCs)* were found to respond less to the HCMV infection than adult dendritic cells. The IL12 and both interferon α and β were produced in lower amounts by cord blood DCs that by the adult controls (Renneson et al. 2009). Acute maternal cytomegalovirus infection was found to be associated with significantly decreased numbers of CD34+ cells in umbilical cord blood (Jaime-Pérez et al. 2012).

The number of dendritic cells (DCs) and the function of plasmacytoid DCs (pDC) were similar between subjects and controls and were not correlated with maternal or neonatal *hepatitis B viremia* (Koumbi et al. 2010).

The U83 protein of *human herpesvirus 6 (HHV-6)* is able to bind a series of chemokine receptors. Virus-coded U3 protein of HHV-6B appears to be restricted to CCR2 signaling, whereas the U83 from HHV-6A binds with high affinity and activates CCR1, CCR4, CCR5, CCR6, and CCR8 (Dewin et al. 2006; Catusse et al. 2007). HHV-6 also encodes two chemokine receptors,

U12 and U51. Expression of U51 can be prevented *in vitro* by siRNA. The reduced replication of HHV-6 suggests that U51 plays an essential role for viral growth (Catusse et al. 2008).

The U24 expression of HHV-6 causes internalization of the T cell receptor/CD3 complex at the cell surface, resulting in improper T cell activation by antigen-presenting cells (Sullivan and Coscoy, 2008).

The HHV-6 carrier state was found to be a trigger, for acute graft versus host disease (aGvHD) in bone marrow transplant recipients. The HHV-6 reactivation before the first 120 days of transplantation was found to be significantly more frequent (3.2) in the case of those who obtained cord blood cells and in the patients treated with cells of unrelated donors. The post transplantation screening of the recipients after UCB transplantation was recommended only in the case of clinical symptoms in order to make specific chemotherapy possible (Appleton et al. 1995; Betts et al. 2011; Pichereau et al. 2012). Free viral HHV-6 DNA has been detected in the cord blood and saliva of non-ciHHV-6-carrier children born to ciHHV-6 mothers, suggesting the possibility of transplacental transmission of free virus (Hall et al. 2010; Reviewed by Pellett et al. 2012

Prenatal human parvovirus B19 infection can prime fetal B cells and fetal IgM can be detected in the cord blood samples of every fourth newborn (Weiffenbach et al. 2012).

HCV-exposed neonates had significantly lower levels of regulatory T cells expressing HLA-DR, lower CD4+ and CD8+ T cell activation, and lower plasma levels of pro-inflammatory markers than did controls. However, CD4+ and CD8+ T cells from HCV-exposed neonates had higher IFN-γ production in response to polyclonal stimulation than did T cells from controls (Babik et al. 2011). HCV exposure had multiple effects on cord blood cells including a decrease in activation markers (CD69, TRAIL and NKp44) on NK cells and a decrease in plasmacytoid dendritic cells in both placenta and cord blood of exposed infants (Hurtado et al. 2010).

Influenza A induced dose-dependent apoptosis of NK cells with down-regulation of NKp46 expression, which was more pronounced in UCB (Lin et al. 2012).

In vitro experiments have revealed, that fetal priming of memory T-cells to exogenous antigens enhances specific proviral gene transcription pathways in effector memory cells that may increase risk of vertical transmission of HIV (Steiner et al. 2010, 2012). The expression pattern of the neonatal mononuclear cells was shown to influence the replication of the HIV (Sundaravaradan et al. 2010).

Severe *respiratory syncytium virus (RSV)* diseases were preceded by the significant downregulation of Dicer mRNA production of cord blood cells probably responsible for the severty of the clinical appearence (Inchley et al. 2011). A wide range of antiviral responses in cord blood monocytes across the population and the decrease in production of IFN-γ (but not CCL5) mRNA in response to respiratory syncytial virus infection of cord blood monocytes *in vitro* was found to be associated with a significant increase in the frequency of upper respiratory tract infections and the prevalence of ear and sinus infections, pneumonias, and respiratory-related hospitalizations in the first year of life. The viruses detected were: *Rhinoviruses, Adenoviruses, RSV, Coronaviruses, Enteroviruses, Parainfluenza virus, Influenzavirus, Metapneumovirus, Bocavirus and multiple viruses* (Sumino et al. 2012).

Mast cells are innate immune cells that play a sentinel cell role in host protection against infectious agents via pathogen-recognition receptors by producing potent mediators that modulate inflammation, cell recruitment and normal vascular homeostasis. Mast cells are connective tissue-associated leukocytes located at areas of external interface, such as the skin and mucous membranes.

Mast cells are susceptible to antibody enhanced *dengue virus infection* and respond with selective cytokine and chemokine responses. Activate human endothelial cells, as evidenced by increased expression of the adhesion molecules ICAM-1 and VCAM-1. Dengue virus infection of human mast cells is antibody dependent, leading to TNF production. Antibody-virus complexes bind through FcγRIIs to the cells. In order to obtain a global view of dengue virus-induced gene regulation in mast cells, primary human cord blood-derived mast cells were tested and were identified as representing an important source of TNF (Brown et al. 2006, 2011).

In order to accelerate antigen presentation and intercellular costimulation have been suggested for the *ex vivo* priming of antigen-specific T cells. IL-7, IL-15, and IL-12 decrease the antigen concentration threshold, direct T cells toward a central memory phenotype, and influence the polarization of T8+ cytotoxic type 1 and T4+ helper type 1 cells. In combination these cytokines augment the generation of antigen-specific CTLs from naive T cells combined with recombinant adenovirus priming and Epstein-Barr virus transformation (Hanley et al. 2009, 2012).

Enveloped virus but not bacteria block IL-13 responses in human cord blood T cells (Svensson et al. 2012).

Maternal Fetal Microchymerism and the Cord Blood Cells

The definition of maternal-fetal microchimerism is the transfer of maternal cells to the offspring. Maternal hematopoietic and nonhematopoietic cells were shown to persist into adulthood (van Halteren et al. 2009). Maternal cells enter the fetal circulation first and are capable of migration to fetal and neonatal organs. This is of importance with regard to potential consequences of umbilical cord blood transplantation and postnatal development of autoimmune disease (Srivatsa et al. 2003). The placenta prevents the transfer of malignant cells into the fetal organism (Hörmann and Lentis, 1965; van Rood et al. 2012). In spite of this, among the maternal cells in the cord blood might be premalignant and malignant cells (Reviewed by Berencsi and Barcsay, 2012).

The prerequisite of the survival of the transfered cells in the foreign organism is the phenomenon of actively acquired tolerance developping in the acceptor organism (Billingham et al. 1953).

Transgenerational Immune-Modulation

The *antibody network theory* has been published in 1974 (Jerne, 1974). As early as in 1989 it has been observed, that induction of lysis via CD2 shows qualitatively different activation requirements in T cell receptor (TCR) gamma+ delta+/CD3+, TCR alpha beta+/CD3+ CTL and TCR-/CD3- NK cells (Goedegebuure et al. 1989). Cytotoxic T lymphocyte activation was shown to occur via CD16 and it was regulated by CD3 and CD8 antigens. Studies with T cell receptor (TCR)-alpha beta+/CD3+16+ and TCR-gamma delta+/CD3+16+ granular lymphocytes (Oshimi et al 1990). It has been shown, that an antigen specific T-helper signal and IL4 are required for the production of specific antibodies by B-cells (Guy and Hodes, 1989).

It has been suggested in 1990, that part of the *therapeutic effects of intravenous immunoglobulin (IVIg)* infusion, might be mediated through idiotype/antiidiotype interactions (Carreras et al. 1990) and due to interaction of antibodies with B- and T-cell receptors (Rudensky et al. 1990). Transplacental IgG is also able to participate in such interactions with both B- and T-cells.

Kidney transplant recipients, who had been treated with TCR-complex (OKT3) specific therapy to prevent rejection developed two types of anti-OKT3 *(anti-idiotypic antibodies) alpha and beta* (Carreno et al. 1992).

Multitransfused patients were found to develop *antibody against T-cell receptor (TCR).* It was suggested that the TCR antibody binds to TCR of the T-cell clones, thus blocking the interaction of the T-cell clone with alloantigens of stimulator cells and resulting in inhibition of the proliferation of T-cell clones. On the basis of the T-cell clone-specific binding of the antibody in sera, it has been concluded that the antibody was anti-idiotypic (Nishimura et al. 1992). The possible role of anti-idiotype antibodies (Ab2) has been reviewed by McIntyre (1992). The role of anti-idiotype antibody as blocking antibodies in the serum responsible for infertility has been suggested by Yagami in 1993 (Yagami, 1993).

Maternal immunization was shown to modify the immune response of mice against 2-o-phenyl-oxasolon (Lemke et al. 1994).

The *antigenic mimicry* of the molecular differences between the variable regions of antibodies and anti-idiotypes has been also clarified (Fields et al. 1995).

Anti-idiotype antibodies were found to regulate the production of complementary antibodies (Borghesi and Nicoletti, 1996).

In mice with experimental anti-phospholipid syndrome (APS), maternal anti-Id effect was associated with a rise in the number of IL-2 and interferon-gamma (IFN-g)-secreting cells (Th1) and reduction in IL-4- and IL-6-secreting cells (Th2) i.e. activation of DC, CD8 and Th1 and Th2 cells (Krause et al. 1999).

The *maternally induced imprinting* was suggested by Lemke and Lange (1999). Generalization of single immunological experiences by idiotypically mediated clonal connections (Lemke and Lange, 2002). Leading to the theory of Lamarkian inheritance by somatically acquired IgG phenotypes (Lemke et al. 2004).

Active immunization could be achieved even against bacterial infections using anti-idiotypic IgG (Beninati et al. 2001). Maternal autoantibody triggers *de novo* T cell-mediated neonatal autoimmune disease (Setiady et al. 2003). The transplacental transmission of maternal autoantibodies in many patients results in *transient neonatal illnesses* (Reviewed recently by Berencsi and Szomor, 2012). The concentration of anti-idiotypes in maternal serum can mitigate the severity of the neonatal illness (Setiady et al. 2003; Stea et al. 2006).

Anti-idiotype antibodies have been identified in patients suffering from multiple sclerosis which were complementary to oxidized phosphatidylcholine [1-palmitoyl-2-(5'-oxo)valeryl-sn-glycero-3-phosphorylcholine (Qin et al.

2007). The production of anti-idiotype antibodies by umbilical cord B-cells has been shown, too (Warrington et al. 1995).

The newborns of mothers vaccinated with subunit influenza vaccines produced IgM-type antibodies to matrix proteins of the virus (about 40 %) and sensitized T-lymphocytes even in such persons, who's HLA-type was of paternal origin. This later finding excluded the role of maternal-fetal microchymerism in the transfer of cells. The second result excluding the role of microchymerism was the fact that no IgM could be detected in several maternal sera, who's cord blood was positive for fetal IgM (Rastogi et al. 2007).

According to the oppinion of the authors of this chapter the transplacental transfer of maternal anti-idiotypes might be responsible for the priming of fetal B and T cells. The overhelming majority of efficacy tests of influenza vaccination are performed using hemagglutination inhibition (HAI) tests, and therefore no data are available on the specific IgM content of the cord blood (Heiny et al, 2007; Tan et al. 2010; Tsatsaris et al. 2011; Fisher et al. 2012; Lin et al. 2012). The matrix protein specific antibodies cannot be measured by HAI test, therefore the production of specific IgM became obvious (Rastogi et al. 2007). Maternally-mediated immunological imprinting has been experimentally documented by Lemke et al. (2009). Allergen IgE-isotype-specific suppression by maternally derived monoclonal anti-IgG-idiotype was also shown (Tanasa et al. 2010) and the whole topic of *transgenerational messengers* has been reviewed by Lemke et al. (2012). Antibody copies of regulatory peptides (anti-idiotypes) could be used for the treatment of influenzavirus infections (Conti et al. 2008). Both idiotype (Ab1) and anti-idiotype antibodies (Ab2) were found to interact with T-cell receptors (TCRs) and participate in T-cell regulation (Martinez et al. 1986a and b; Jacobsen et al. 2010). Chimeric IgG1 version of a polyreactive α anti-idiotype antibody that is able to interact with different immunoglobulins and non-immunoglobulin antigens. The formation of immune complexes seems to be necessary, but not sufficient, to this activity. The potential immunostimulating effect involving of the interaction of the anti-idiotype B7Y33 MAB with the FcγRIIb is discussed (Hernández et al. 2012). Recently antibody maturation intermediates that are related to broadly neutralizing antibodies (bnAbs) against the HIV-1 and other viruses have been identified as observed in normal individuals, and compared their genetic diversity and somatic mutation level along with available structural and functional data. Most of the germline subgroups were identified with frequencies comparable to those present in the adult IgM repertoire except for the IGHV1-2 gene that was preferentially expressed in the cord blood cells. Human cord blood antibody repertoires, which have gene usage diversity and VHCDR3 lengths similar to that of the adult IgM repertoire but differ significantly in some of the gene usages, V-D-J rearrangements, junctional diversity, and somatic mutations (Prabakaran et al. 2012a and b). One child showed positive IgM in fetal blood (FB) but developed normally. The mother suffered from Varicella-Zoster 20 weeks preceeding pregnancy! This also might be an indication for the immunizing effect of transplacental VZV-specific anti-idiotype (Ab2). The asymptomatic infected child grew healthy until the completion of screening tests when it reached 5 years old (Sanchez et al. 2011). Two types of enzymes play a key role in Ab diverseness, i. e., the products of recombination-activating genes RAG1 and RAG2 and the affinity induced deaminase (AID) (Reviewed by Mix et al. 2006). A small portion of the IgG circulating in the fetus expressed a non-maternal haplotype. Umbilical endothelial cells were shown to be capable of synthesizing IgG with properties similar to those of immune cells and that they may play additional roles besides lining the vessels and transporting IgG. RAG1 (recombination activating gene 1), RAG2, and variable (V), diversity (D), and joining (J) segments for recombination of IgG, were also found in these cells by RT-PCR and realtime PCR. These results indicate that *umbilical endothelial cells are capable of synthesizing IgG* with properties similar to those of immune cells and that they may play additional roles besides lining the vessels and transporting IgG. The presence of IgG at the mRNA level in trophoblasts, strongly indicated that such cells can produce IgG, too (Zhao et al. 2011).

Influence of External Circumstances on Reactivation of Latent Viruses

The presence of tumour-promoter substances in food (phorbiates from *Euphorbia* plants) consumed in far-eastern countries has been suggested as cofactors facilitating the development of nasopharingeal cancer (Gschwendt and Hecker, 1969, 1973). The role of *Eptein-Barr virus (EBV)* in the etiology of nasopharingeal carcinoma has been reviewed the same time (Ho, 1972). The possible effect of smoking, radioactive substances of food origin and seal oil lamps of Eskimos has been analysed (Schaefer et al. 1975). The EBV-specific antibodies have been tested of Eskimos before the development of nasopharingeal cacinoma and no difference could be found in comparison to the healthy controls.

As early as in 1977 de-Thé in Lyon suggested, that the week immune response due to perinatal EBV infection might be responsible for the development of Burkitt's lymphoma. All children suffering from *Burkitt's lymphoma* proved to be seropositive at 6 months of age (de-Thé, 1977). The significant increase of specific antibodies could be observed several months before the onset of the disease (Lanier et al. 1980, 1989). In contrast to the findings of de-Thé in the tropical belt of Africa, where an impaired immune response was observed in the 6 months old babies (de-Thé, 1977). When the presence of EBV became evident in 4 % of the amniotic fluids at term of healthy newborns, the idea has been put foreward, that the immunomodulation could be even more expressed following transplacental infection (Younes et al. 2007, 2009).

Women with depression have higher prevalence of Epstein-Barr virus reactivation, possibly due to increased stress. The EBV reactivation occurred in the case of every 3rd pregnant and the reactivation occurred mainly in the 2nd trimester (Haeri et al. 2010, 2011).

It was shown recently, that exposure of the Epstein-Barr virus carrier cells to *Euphorbia tirucali* extract has been able to reactivate EBV and cause chromosomal alterations, which leads to altered expression of c-MYC also in cells of cord blood origin facilitating polyploidity (Mannucci et al. 2012).

Cord blood cells taken from children of *family history of allergy* expressed epsilon-specific mRNA and mRNA for interleukin-2 (IL-2), IL-4, IL-10 and interferon-gamma (IFN-gamma) but not IL-6. At 7 months of age, peripheral blood mononuclear cells expressed epsilon-specific mRNA and mRNA for all cytokines. In the placental membrane, IgE+ cells, while CD8+CD60+ T cells were detected in the chorionic villi. CD8+CD60+ T cells, cells expressing epsilon-specific and IL-6-specific mRNA might contribute to the pathobiology and provide important prognostic indicators of atopy. Immunoglobulin levels were within normal ranges and IgE levels were negligible in cord blood and at 7 months of age (Smith-Norowitz et al. 2008).

Possible Algorithms for Surveillance of Viruses Present in the Cord Blood Samples

Lymphotrop herpesviruses (EBV, HCMV, HHV-6, HHV-7 and HHV-8) using PCR of amniotic fluid at delivery (Younes et al. 2007). Differentiation of integrated and replicating HHV-6 (Caserta et al. 2010; Reviewed by Flamand et al. 2010). HBV, HCV and HIV (López and Coll, 2010).

Retrospective diagnosis of dried cord blood or dried blood spots indicating transplacental transmission of HCMV (Leruez-Ville et al. 2009; Tagawa et al. 2009). Algorithm of HCMV surveillance of low risk pregnants (Peled et al. 2011).

Perspectives of Virus-Free Stem Cell Amplification, Modification and Selection

Graft engineering and modifications of the inner immunological environment of the recipient host by the activation or administration of tumor memory T cells, selected T_{REG} cells and natural killer (NKT) cell classes and cytokines, and the improved pharmacotherapy of GvHD without reducing its antitumor efficacy, will raise the value of GvHD to the higher ranks of the effective antitumor immunotherapeutical measures (Reviewed by Sinkovics, 2010).

Generation of virus-free induced pluripotent stem cell (iPSC) clones from single cells under feeder-free conditions will solve some of the safety concerns related to use of xeno- or allogeneic-material in culture, and contribute to the characterization and the standardization of iPS cells intended for use in a clinical setting (Nishishita et al. 2012). Application of *recombinant viruses* (adenovirus 5/F35) can be used for the examination of the molecular processes that control the development and function of lymphocytes (Samson and Jung, 2011). Lentiviral labeling revealed three germ layer differentiation potential of a single unrestricted somatic stem cell from human cord blood (Wernet et al. 2010).

An extremely potent *HOX-derivative cloned into a lentivirus* that consists of the 50 sequences of a NUP98 cDNA and the homeodomain (*HD)* of the *HOXA10* cDNA termed NA10HD enabled a subsequent rapid and marked expansion *in vitro* of mouse hematopoietic stem cell numbers without causing their transformation or deregulated expansion *in vivo*. (Sloma et al. 2012).

References

Aaskov JG, Nair K, Lawrence GW, Dalglish DA, Tucker M.: Evidence for transplacental transmission of Ross River virus in humans. *Med. J. Aust.* 1981; 2: 20-1.

Acs N, Banhidy F, Puho E, Czeizel AE.: Maternal influenza during pregnancy and risk of congenital abnormalities in offspring. Birth Defects Res Part A *Clin. Mol. Teratol.* 2005; 73: 989–96.

Adler SP.: Screening for cytomegalovirus during pregnancy. *Infect Dis. Obstet Gynecol.* 2011; 2011:1-9.

Adorini L, Penna G, Giarratana N, Uskokovic M.: Tolerogenic dendritic cells induced by vitamin D receptor ligands enhance regulatory T cells inhibiting allograft rejection and autoimmune diseases. *J. Cell Biochem.* 2003; 88: 227–33.

Adams LL, Gungor S, Turan S, Kopelman JN, Harman CR, Baschat AA.: When are amniotic fluid viral PCR studies indicated in prenatal diagnosis? When are amniotic fluid viral PCR studies indicated in prenatal diagnosis? *Prenat Diagn.* 2012 Jan;32(1):88-93. doi: 10.1002/pd.3835.

Albano MS, Taylor P, Pass RF, Scaradavou A, Ciubotariu R, Carrier C, Dobrila L, Rubinstein P, Stevens CE.: Umbilical cord blood transplantation and cytomegalovirus: Posttransplantation infection and donor screening. *Blood.* 2006; 108: 4275-82.

Al-Hareth Z, Monem F, Abdel Megiud N.: Is low birth weight a risk indicator for congenital cytomegalovirus infection? *J. Infect Dev. Ctries.* 2009; 4: 44-7.

Appleton AL, Sviland L, Peiris JS, Taylor CE, Wilkes J, Green MA, Pearson AD, Kelly PJ, Malcolm AJ, Proctor SJ, et al, for the Newcastle upon Tyne Bone Marrow Transport Group: Humanherpes virus-6 infection in marrow graft recipients: role in pathogenesis of graftversus-host disease. *Bone Marrow Transplant.* 1995; 16: 777-782.

Arbuckle JH, Medveczky MM, Luka J, Hadley SH, Luegmayr A, Ablashi D, Lund TC, Tolar J, De Meirleir K, Montoya JG, Komaroff AL, Ambros PL, Medveczky PG.: The latent human herpesvirus-6A genome specifically integrates in telomeres of human chromosomes in vivo and in vitro, *Proc. Natl. Acad. Sci. USA.* 2010; 107: 5563-8. DOI:10.1073/pnas. 0913586107.

Arbuckle JH, Pantry S, Medveczky PG.: The mechanism and significance of integration and vertical transmission of human herpesvirus 6 genome. In *Maternal fetal transmission of human viruses and their influence on tumorigenesis* pp.171-94. (Ed. Berencsi G III.) Springer, 2012 . DOI: 10.1007/978-94-007-4216-1_5.

Babik JM, Cohan D, Monto A, Hartigan-O'Connor DJ, McCune JM.: The human fetal immune response to hepatitis C virus exposure in utero. *J. Infect Dis.* 2011; 203: 196-206.

Barker JN, Doubrovina E, Sauter C, Jaroscak JJ, Perales MA, Doubrovin M, Prockop SE, Koehne G, O'Reilly RJ.: Successful treatment of EBV-associated posttransplantation lymphoma after cord bloodtransplantation using third-party EBV-specific cytotoxic T lymphocytes. *Blood.* 2010; 116: 5045-9.

Baschat AA, Harman CR, Towbin JA, Weiner CP.: Fetal sonographic abnormalities and intrauterine viral infection. *Am. J. Obstet. Gynecol.* 2000; 182: S95.

Baschat AA, Towbin J, Bowles NE, Harman CR, Weiner CP.: Prevalence of viral DNA in amniotic fluid of low-risk pregnancies in the second trimester. *J. Matern. Fetal. Neonatal Med.* 2003; 13: 381–384.

Belderbos ME, Houben ML, Wilbrink B, Lentjes E, Bloemen EM, Kimpen JL, Rovers M, Bont L.: Cord blood vitamin D deficiency is associated with respiratory syncytial virus bronchiolitis. *Pediatrics.* 2011; 127: e1513-20.

Beninati C, Oggioni M, Mancuso G, Midiri A, Polonelli L, Pozzi G and Teti G.: Anti-idiotypic vaccination against group B streptococci. *Int. Rev. Immunol.* 2001; 20: 263-73. DOI:10.3109/08830180109043038

Berencsi G III and Barcsay E.: Maternal fetal microchimerism and fetal-juvenile malignancies. In *Maternal fetal transmission of human viruses and their influence on tumorigenesis* pp. 335-388. (Ed. Berencsi G III.) Springer, 2012 . DOI: 10.1007/978-94-007-4216-1_10

Berencsi G III and Csire M.: Maternal-fetal infections with human viruses.In *Maternal fetal transmission of human viruses and their influence on tumorigenesis* pp.106-46. (Ed. Berencsi G III.) Springer, 2012 . DOI: 10.1007/978-94-007-4216-1_4

Berencsi György III. and Ördög Katalin: Polarised transfer of proteins through the syncytiotrophobalst and tissue culture cell lines. In *Maternal fetal transmission of human viruses and their influence on tumorigenesis* pp.223-247. (Ed. Berencsi G III.) Springer, 2012. DOI: 10.1007/978-94-007-4216-1_4.

Berencsi, György III and Szomor, Katalin: Fetal and neonatal illnesses caused or influenced by maternal transplacental IgG and/or therapeutic antibodies applied during pregnancy. In *Maternal fetal transmission of human viruses and their influence on tumorigenesis* pp.281-333. (Ed. Berencsi G III.) Springer, 2012. DOI: 10.1007/978-94-007-4216-1_4.

Betts BC, Young JA, Ustun C, Cao Q, Weisdorf DJ.: Human herpesvirus 6 infection after hematopoietic cell transplantation: is routine surveillance necessary? *Biol. Blood Marrow Transplant.* 2011; 17: 1562-8.

Bhat P, Anderson DA.: Hepatitis b virus translocates across a trophoblastic barrier. *J. Virol.* 2007; 81: 7200-7. doi:10.1128/JVI.02371-06.

Bhat Purnima.: Maternal-fetal transmission of HBV. In *Maternal fetal transmission of human viruses and their influence on tumorigenesis* pp. 195-222. (Ed. Berencsi G III.) Springer, 2012. DOI: 10.1007/978-94-007-4216-1_10

Billerbeck E, Kang YH, Walker L, Lockstone H, Grafmueller S, Fleming V, Flint J, Willberg CB, Bengsch B, Seigel B, Ramamurthy N, Zitzmann N, Barnes EJ, Thevanayagam J, Bhagwanani A, Leslie A, Oo YH, Kollnberger S, Bowness P, Drognitz O, Adams DH, Blum HE, Thimme R, Klenerman P.: Analysis of CD161 expression on human CD8+ T cells defines a distinct functional subset with tissue-homing properties. *Proc. Natl. Acad. Sci. USA*. 2010; 107: 3006-11. DOI: 10.1073/pnas.0914839107

Bonvicini F, Puccetti C, Salfi NC, Guerra B, Gallinella G, Rizzo N, Zerbini M.: Gestational and fetal outcomes in B19 maternal infection: a problem of diagnosis. *J. Clin. Microbiol.* 2011; 49: 3514-8. DOI: 10.1128/JCM.00854-11.

Boppana SB, Rivera LB, Fowler KB, Mach M, Britt WJ.: Intrauterine transmission of cytomegalovirus to infants of women with preconceptional immunity. *The New England J. Med.* 2001; 344: 1366–71.

Borghesi C and Nicoletti C.: Autologous anti-idiotypic antibody response is regulated by the level of circulating complementary idiotype. *Immunology*. 1996; 89: 172-7. DOI:10.1046/j.1365-2567.1996.d01-724.x

Bose PD, Das BC, Kumar A, Gondal R, Kumar D, Kar P.: High viral load and deregulation of the progesterone receptor signaling pathway: association with hepatitis E-related poor pregnancy outcome. *J. Hepatol.* 2011; 54: 1107-13.

Bozzo P, Narducci A, Einarson A.: Vaccination during pregnancy. *Can Fam. Physician*. 2011; 57: 555-7.

Brackett BG, Baranska W, Sawicki W, Koprowski H.: Uptake of heterologous genome by mammalian spermatozoa and its transfer to ova through fertilization. *Proc. Natl. Acad. Sci. USA*. 1971; 68: 353-7.

Broccolo F, Drago F, Careddu AM, Foglieni C, Turbino L, Cocuzza CE, Gelmetti C, Lusso P, Rebora AE, Malnati MS.: Additional evidence that pityriasis rosea is associated with reactivation of human herpesvirus-6 and -7. *J. Invest Dermatol.* 2005; 124: 1234-40.

Brown, M. G., C. A. King, C. Sherren, J. S. Marshall, and R. Anderson.: A dominant role for FcgammaRII in antibody-enhanced dengue virus infection of human mast cells and associated CCL5 release. *J. Leukoc. Biol.* 2006; 80: 1242-50.

Brown MG, Hermann LL, Issekutz AC, Marshall JS, Rowter D, Al-Afif A, Anderson R.: Dengue virus infection of mast cells triggers endothelial cell activation. *J. Virol.* 2011; 85: 1145-50. DOI: 10.1128/JVI.01630-10

Burguete T, Rabreau M, Fontanges-Darriet M, Roset E, Hager HD, Koppel A, Bischof P, Schlehofer JR. Evidence for infection of the human embryo with adeno-associated virus in pregnancy. *Hum. Reprod.* 1999; 14: 2396–2401.

Burk RD, Hwang LY, Ho GY, Shafritz DA, Beasley RP.: Outcome of perinatal hepatitis b virus exposure is dependent on maternal virus load. *J. Infect Dis.* 1994; 170: 1418-23. doi:10.1093/infdis/170.6.1418.

Buxmann H, Kamin W, Kriván G, Siklós P, Mendling W, Wartenberg-Demand A, Wolf DM, Schlösser RL.: An open-label, randomized efficacy and safety trial of subcutaneous and intramuscular BT088 (Fovepta) human hepatitis B immunoglobulin in neonates of HBV-carrier mothers. *J. Perinat. Med.* 2012; 40: 433-8. doi: 10.1515/jpm-2011-0185.

Buzzi M, Alviano F, Campioni D, Stignani M, Melchiorri L, Rotola A, Tazzari P, Ricci F, Vaselli C, Terzi A, Pagliaro PP, Cuneo A, Lanza F, Bontadini A, Baricordi OR, Rizzo R.: Umbilical cord blood CD34(+)cell-derived progeny produces human leukocyte antigen-G molecules with immuno-modulatory functions. *Hum. Immunol.* 2012; 73: 150-5.

Canadian Blood Services. Safety and testing. [cited 2011 May 3]. Available from: URL: http://www.bloodservices.ca/CentreApps/Internet/UW_V502_MainEngine.nsf/page/Testing?OpenDocument.

Carreno M, Fuller L, Zucker K, Yang WC, Burke G, Nery J, Gomez C, Esquenazi V, Miller J.: Cross-species reactivity of the anti-idiotype anti-OKT3 cascade between mice and humans. *Hum. Immunol.* 1992; 33: 249-58.

Carreras LO, Pérez GN, Martinuzzo ME, Malan-Borel I, Malbrán A, Said PB.: Partial neutralization of a lupus anticoagulant by human immunoglobulin. *Thromb Haemost.* 1990; 64: 32-7.

Caserta MT, Hall CB, Schnabel K, Lofthus G, Marino A, Shelley L, Yoo C, Carnahan J, Anderson L, Wang H.: Diagnostic assays for active infection with human herpesvirus 6 (HHV-6). *J. Clin. Virol.* 2010; 48: 55-7. DOI::10.1016/j.jcv.2010.02.007.

Cason J, Rice P, Best JM.: Transmission of cervical cancerassociated human papilloma viruses from mother to child. *Intervirol* 1998; 41:213–218.

Catusse J, Parry CM, Dewin DR, Gompels UA.: Inhibition of HIV-1 infection by viral chemokine U83A via high-affinity CCR5 interactions that block human chemokine-induced leukocyte chemotaxis and receptor internalization. *Blood* 2007; 109: 3633–9.

Catusse J, Spinks J, Mattick C, Dyer A, Laing K, Fitzsimons C, Smit MJ, Gompels UA.: Immunomodulation by herpesvirus U51A chemokine receptor via CCL5 and FOG-2 down-regulation plus XCR1 and CCR7 mimicry in human leukocytes. *Eur. J. Immunol* 2008; 38: 763–77.

CDC-Centers for Disease Control and Prevention.: Intrauterine West Nile virus infection--New York, 2002. *MMWR Morb Mortal Wkly Rep*. 2002; 51: 1135-6.

CDC-Centers for Disease Control and Prevention .: Possible congenital infection with La Crosse encephalitis virus--West Virginia, 2006-2007. *MMWR Morb. Mortal Wkly Rep*. 2009; 58: 4-7.

Chamberland ME, Alter HJ, Busch MP, Nemo G, Ricketts M.: Emerging infectious disease issues in blood safety. *Emerg. Infect Dis*. 2001; 7 Suppl: 552-3.

Chaturvedi UC, Mathur A, Chandra A, Das SK, Tandon HO, Singh UK.: Transplacental infection with Japanese encephalitis virus. *J. Infect. Dis*. 1980; 141: 712-5. DOI: 10.1093/infdis/141.6.712.

Chen AC, Keleher A, Kedda MA, Spurdle AB, McMillan NA, Antonsson A.: Human papillomavirus DNA detected in peripheral blood samples from healthy Australian maleblood donors. *J. Med. Virol*. 2009; 81: 1792-6.

Chen AY, Guan W, Lou S, Liu Z, Kleiboeker S, Qiu J.: Role of erythropoietin receptor signaling in parvovirus B19 replication in human erythroid progenitor cells. *J. Virol*. 2010; 84: 12385-96.

Chen AY, Zhang EY, Guan W, Cheng F, Kleiboeker S, Yankee TM, Qiu J.: The small 11 kDa nonstructural protein of human parvovirus B19 plays a key role in inducing apoptosis during B19 virus infection of primary erythroid progenitor cells. *Blood*. 2010; 115: 1070-80.

Chen AY, Kleiboeker S, Qiu J.: Productive parvovirus B19 infection of primary humanerythroid progenitor cells at hypoxia is regulated by STAT5A and MEK signaling but not HIFα. *PLoS Pathog*. 2011; 7: e1002088.

Chen W, Streaker ED, Russ DE, Feng Y, Prabakaran P, Dimitrov DS.: Characterization of germline antibody libraries from human umbilical cord blood and selection of monoclonal antibodies to viral envelope glycoproteins: Implications for mechanisms of immune evasion and design of vaccine immunogens. *Biochem. Biophys. Res. Commun.* 2012; 417: 1164-9.

Coleman CB, Nealy MS, Tibbetts SA.: Immature and transitional B cells are latency reservoirs for a gammaherpesvirus. *J. Virol.* 2010; 84: 13045-52.

Concato C, Diociaiuti A, Parisi F, Giraldi L, Ciasulli A, Menichella D, El Hachem M.: Human herpesvirus-8 serology in pediatric organ transplantation. *Transplant Proc.* 2008; 40: 3683-4.

Conti G, Magliani W, Conti S, Nencioni L, Sgarbanti R, Palamara AT and Polonelli L.: Therapeutic activity of an anti-idiotypic antibody-derived killer peptide against influenza A virus experimental infection. *Antimicrob. Agents Chemother.* 2008; 52: 4331-7. DOI:10.1128/ AAC.00506-08

Coppoletta S, Tedone E, Galano B, Soracco M, Raiola AM, Lamparelli T, Gualandi F, Bregante S, Ibatici A, di Grazia C, Dominietto A, Varaldo R, Bruno B, Frassoni F, Van Lint MT, Bacigalupo A.: *Biol. Blood Marrow Transplant.* 2011; 17: 901-7.

Cotmore SF, Tattersall P.: A rolling-haipin strategy: basic mechanisms of DNA replication in the parvoviruses. pp 171–181. In: Kerr J, Cotmore SF, Bloom ME, Linden RM, Parrish CR, eds. *Parvoviruses.* 2005; London: Hoddler Arond.

Couzi L, Pitard V, Sicard X, Garrigue I, Hawchar O, Merville P, Moreau JF, Déchanet-Merville J.: Antibody-dependent anti-cytomegalovirus activity of human γδ T cells expressing CD16 (FcγRIIIa). *Blood.* 2012; 119: 1418-27.

Csire M, Mikala G, Jákó J, Masszi T, Jánosi J, Dolgos J, Füle T, Tordai A, Berencsi G, Vályi-Nagy I.: Persistent long-term human herpesvirus 6 (HHV-6) infection in a patient with langerhans cell histiocytosis. *Pathol. Oncol. Res.* 2007; 13: 157-60.

Csire M, Mikala G, Pető M, Jánosi J, Juhász A, Tordai A, Jákó J, Domján Gy, Dolgos J, Berencsi G, Vályi-Nagy I.: Detection of four lymphotropic herpesviruses inHungarian Patients with multiplemyeloma and lymphoma. *FEMS Immunol. Med. Microbiol* 2007; 49: 62–67 DOI:10.1111/j.1574-695X.2006.00171.x

Csire M, Mikala G.: Human herpesviruses in hematologic diseases. In *Herpesviridae* 107-36 (Eds. Magel GD, Tyring S), Intech 2012.

Czeglédy J., Gergely L., Endrodi I.: Detection of human papillomavirus deoxyribonucleic acid by filter in situ hybridization during pregnancy. *J. Med. Virol.* 28: 250-4. (1989). DOI:10.1002/jmv.1890280409.

Czegledy J.: Sexual and non-sexual transmission of human papillomavirus. Acta Microbiol Immunol Hung 2001; 48: 511–517

de Jong EP, Walther FJ, Kroes AC, Oepkes D.: Parvovirus B19 infection in pregnancy: new insights and management. *Prenat Diagn.* 2011; 31: 419-25. DOI: 10.1002/pd.2714.

Delage G, Carter AO.: Hepatitis B Infection in Canada: Epidemiology and implications for control. *Can. Fam. Physician.* 1992; 38: 2656-8, 2661-2, 2665-6.

de Pagter PJ, Virgili A, Nacheva E, van Baarle D, Schuurman R, Boelens JJ.: Chromosomally integrated human herpesvirus 6: transmission via cord blood-derived unrelated hematopoietic stem cell transplantation. *Biol. Blood Marrow Transplant.* 2010; 16: 130-2.

De Paschale M, Agrappi C, Manco MT, Paganini A, Clerici P.: Incidence and risk of Cytomegalovirus infection during pregnancy in an urban area of northern Italy. *Infect Dis Obstet Gynecol.* 2009; 1-5. doi:10.1155/2009/206505.

de-The G.: Is Burkitt's lymphoma related to perinatal infection by Epstein-Barr virus? Lancet. 1977; 1: 335-8. doi:10.1016/S0140-6736(77)91137-0.

Dewin DR, Catusse J, Gompels UA.: Identification and characterization of U83A viral chemokine, a broad and potent beta-chemokine agonist for human CCRs with unique selectivity and inhibition by spliced isoform. *J. Immunol.* 2006; 176: 544–556.

Dencs A, Hettmann A, Szomor KN, Kis Z, Takács M.: Prevalence and genotyping of group 3 torque teno viruses detected in health care workers in Hungary. *Virus Genes.* 2009; 39: 39-45.

Denzer K, Kleijmeer MJ, Heijnen HF, Stoorvogel W, Geuze HJ.: Exosome: from internal vesicle of the multivesicular body to intercellular signaling device. *J. Cell Sci.* 2000; 113: 3365–74.

Diomede L, Nyoka S, Pastori C, Scotti L, Zambon A, Sherman G, Gray CM, Sarzotti-Kelsoe M, Lopalco L.: Passively transmitted gp41 antibodies in babies born from HIV-1 subtype C-seropositive women: correlation between fine specificity and protection. *J. Virol.* 2012; 86: 4129-38.

Domínguez MC, Torres M, Tamayo O, Criollo W, Quintana M, Sánchez A, García F.: [Autoimmune syndrome in the tropical spastic paraparesis/myelopathy associated with human T-lymphotropic virus infections]. *Biomedica.* 2008; 28: 510-22. Spanish.

Drago F, Broccolo F, Zaccaria E, Malnati M, Cocuzza C, Lusso P, Rebora A.: Pregnancy outcome in patients with pityriasis rosea. *J. Am. Acad. Dermatol.* 2008; 58(5 Suppl 1): S78-83.

Drago F, Broccolo F, Rebora A.: Pityriasis rosea: an update with a critical appraisal of its possible herpesviral etiology. *J. Am. Acad. Dermatol.* 2009; 61: 303-18. Review.

Dupuy S, Lambert M, Zucman D, Choukem SP, Tognarelli S, Pages C, Lebbé C, Caillat-Zucman S.: Human Herpesvirus 8 (HHV8) sequentially shapes the NK cell repertoire during the course of asymptomatic infection and Kaposi sarcoma. *PLoS Pathog*. 2012 Jan; 8(1): e1002486.

El-Cheikh J, Fürst S, Casalonga F, Crocchiolo R, Castagna L, Granata A, Oudin C, Faucher C, Berger P, Sarran A, Blaise D.: JC Virus Leuko-Encephalopathy in Reduced Intensity Conditioning Cord Blood Transplant Recipient with a Review of the Literature. *Mediterr J. Hematol Infect Dis*. 2012; 4: e2012043.

El-Sageyer MM, Szenrői A, Hütter E, Új M, Szűcs G, Mezey I, Tóth I, Kátai A, Kapiller Z, Páll G, Petrás G, Szalay E, Mihály I, Gourova S, Berencsi G: Characterization of an epidemic echovirus 11' (prime) epidemic strain causing haemorrhagic hepatitis among newborn babies in Hungary. *Acta virol* 1998; 42: 157-66.

Enders M, Helbig S, Hunjet A, Pfister H, Reichhuber C, Motz M.: Comparative evaluation of two commercial enzyme immunoassays for serodiagnosis of human parvovirus B19 infection. *J. Virol Methods*. 2007; 146: 409-13.

Enders G, Daiminger A, Bäder U, Exler S, Enders M.: Intrauterine transmission and clinical outcome of 248 pregnancies with primary cytomegalovirus infection in relation to gestational age. *J. Clin. Virol.* 2011; 52: 244-6.

Fields BA, Goldbaum FA, Ysern X, Poljak RJ, Mariuzza RA.: Molecular basis of antigen mimicry by an anti-idiotope. *Nature*. 1995; 374: 739-42. DOI:10.1038/374739a0.

Fisher BM, Van Bockern J, Hart J, Lynch AM, Winn VD, Gibbs RS, Weinberg A.: Pandemic influenza A H1N1 2009 infection versus vaccination: a cohort study comparing immune responses in pregnancy. *PLoS One*. 2012; 7(3): e33048.

Flamand L, Komaroff AL, Arbuckle JH, Medveczky PG, Ablashi DV.: Review, part 1: Human herpesvirus-6-basic biology, diagnostic testing, and antiviral efficacy. *J. Med. Virol*. 2010; 82: 1560-8. Review.

Foresta C, Garolla A, Zuccarello D, Pizzol D, Moretti A, Barzon L, Palù G.: Human papillomavirus found in sperm head of young adult males affects the progressive motility. *Fertil Steril*. 2010; 93: 802-6. DOI:10.1016/j.fertnstert.2008.10.050.

Foresta C, Patassini C, Bertoldo A, Menegazzo M, Francavilla F, Barzon L, Ferlin A.: Mechanism of human papillomavirus binding to human spermatozoa and fertilizing ability of infected spermatozoa. PLoS One. 2011 Mar 7; 6(3): e15036. DOI:10.1371/journal.pone.0015036

Foresta C, Ferlin A, Bertoldo A, Patassini C, Zuccarello D, Garolla A.: Human papilloma virus in the sperm cryobank: an emerging problem? Int J Androl. 2011; 34: 242-6. DOI: 10.1111/j.1365-2605.2010.01075.x.

Fowler KB, Stagno S, Pass RF, Britt WJ, Boll TJ, Alford CA.: The outcome of congenital cytomegalovirus infection in relation to maternal antibody status. *The New Engl J. Med.* 1992; 326: 663–7.

Fowler KB, Stagno S, Pass RF.: Maternal immunity and prevention of congenital cytomegalovirus infection. *J. Amer Med. Assoc* 2003; 289: 1008–11.

Gagneur A, Dirson E, Audebert S, Vallet S, Legrand-Quillien MC, Laurent Y, Collet M, Sizun J, Oger E, Payan C.: Materno-fetal transmission of human coronaviruses: a prospective pilot study. *Eur. J. Clin. Microbiol. Infect* Dis. 2008; 27: 863-6.

George B, Pati N, Gilroy N, Ratnamohan M, Huang G, Kerridge I, Hertzberg M, Gottlieb D, Bradstock K.: Pre-transplant cytomegalovirus (CMV) serostatus remains the most important determinant of CMV reactivation after allogeneic hematopoietic stem cell transplantation in the era of surveillance and preemptive therapy. *Transpl Infect Dis.* 2010; 12: 322-9. DOI: 10.1111/j.1399-3062.2010.00504.x.

Gerardin P , Barau G , Michault A , Bintner M , Randrianaivo H , Choker G , Lenglet Y , Touret Y , Bouveret A , Grivard P , Le Roux K , Blanc S , Schuffenecker I , Couderc T , Arenzana-Seisdedos F , Lecuit M , Robillard PY.: Multidisciplinary prospective study of mother-to-child Chikungunya virus infections on the island of La Reunion. *PLoS Med* 2008; 5: e60.

Gervasi MT, Romero R, Bracalente G, Chaiworapongsa T, Erez O, Dong Z, Hassan SS, Yeo L, Yoon BH, Mor G, Barzon L, Franchin E, Militello V, Palù G.: Viral invasion of the amniotic cavity (VIAC) in the midtrimester of pregnancy. *J. Matern Fetal. Neonatal Med.* 2012 May 30. DOI: 10.3109/14767058.2012.683899.

Goedegebuure PS, Segal DM, Braakman E, Vreugdenhil RJ, Van Krimpen BA, Van de Griend RJ, Bolhuis RL.: Induction of lysis by T cell receptor gamma delta+/CD3+ T lymphocytes via CD2 requires triggering via the T11.1 epitope only. *J. Immunol.* 1989; 142: 1797-802.

Gold DR, Bloomberg GR, Cruikshank WW, Visness CM, Schwarz J, Kattan M, O'Connor GT, Wood RA, Burger MS, Wright RJ, Witter F, Lee-Parritz A, Sperling R, Sadovsky Y, Togias A, Gern JE.: Parental characteristics, somatic fetal growth, and season of birth influence innate and adaptive cord blood cytokine responses. *J. Allergy Clin. Immunol.* 2009; 124: 1078-87.

Gschwendt M, Hecker E.: Tumor promoting compounds from Euphorbia triangularis: mono- and diesters of 12-desoxy-phorbol. *Tetrahedron Lett.* 1969; 40: 3509-12.

Gschwendt M, Hecker E.: [On the biologically active compounds of euphorbiaceae. I. Skinirritant and cocarcinogenic factors from Euphorbia cooperi N.E.Br (author's transl)]. *Z Krebsforsch Klin Onkol. Cancer Res. Clin Oncol.* 1973; 80: 335-50. German.

Guy R, Hodes RJ.: Antigen-specific, MHC-restricted B cell activation by cell-free Th2 cell products. Synergy between antigen-specific helper factors and IL-4. *J. Immunol.* 1989; 143: 1433-40.

Haeri S, Baker AM, Boggess KA.: Prevalence of Epstein-Barr virus reactivation in pregnancy. *Am. J. Perinatol.* 2010; 27: 715-9.

Haeri S, Johnson N, Baker AM, Stuebe AM, Raines C, Barrow DA, Boggess KA.: Maternal depression and Epstein-Barr virus reactivation in early pregnancy. *Obstet Gynecol.* 2011; 117(4):862-6.

Heiny AT, Miotto O, Srinivasan KN, Khan AM, Zhang GL, Brusic V, Tan TW, August JT.:Evolutionarily conserved protein sequences of influenza a viruses, avian and human, as vaccine targets. *PLoS ONE* 2007; 2: e1190.

Hall CB, Caserta MT, Schnabel KC, Shelley LM, Carnahan JA, Marino AS, Yoo C, Lofthus GK.: Transplacental congenital human herpesvirus 6 infection caused by maternal chromosomally integrated virus. *J. Infect Dis.* 2010; 201: 505-7.

Hanley PJ, Cruz CR, Savoldo B, Leen AM, Stanojevic M, Khalil M, Decker W, Molldrem JJ, Liu H, Gee AP, Rooney CM, Heslop HE, Dotti G, Brenner MK, Shpall EJ, Bollard CM.: Functionally active virus-specific T cells that target CMV, adenovirus, and EBV can be expanded from naive T-cell populations in cord blood and will target a range of viral epitopes. *Blood.* 2009; 114: 1958-67.

Hanley PJ, Lam S, Shpall EJ, Bollard CM.: Expanding cytotoxic T lymphocytes from umbilical cord blood that target cytomegalovirus, Epstein-Barr virus, and adenovirus. *J. Vis. Exp.* 2012; 63: e3627. DOI: 10.3791/3627.

Hema-Québec.: Safety measures in place. [cited 2011 May 24]. Available from: URL: http://www.hema-quebec.qc.ca/comprendre/mesures-de-securite/securite-enplace. en.html.

Hernández T, Mateo de Acosta C, Pérez R.: Immunopotentiating properties of a multispecific α-anti-idiotype antibody. *MAbs.* 2012 May 1; 4(3).

Ho JHC: Nasopharyngeal carcinoma. *Adv. Cancer Res.* 1972; 15: 57-72.

Hofmann J, Führer A, Bolz M, Waldschläger-Terpe J, Meier M, Lüdders D, Enders M, Oltmann A, Meisel H, Krüger DH.: Hantavirus infections by Puumala or Dobrava-Belgrade virus in pregnant women. *J. Clin. Virol.* 2012 Aug 6.

Holder BS, Tower CL, Forbes K, Mulla MJ, Aplin JD, Abrahams VM.: Immune cell activation by trophoblast-derived microvesicles is mediated by syncytin 1. *Immunology.* 2012; 136: 184-91. DOI: 10.1111/j.1365-2567.2012.03568.x.

Holder BS, Tower CL, Jones CJ, Aplin JD, Abrahams VM.: Heightened pro-inflammatory effect of preeclamptic placental microvesicles on peripheral blood immune cells in humans. *Biol Reprod.* 2012; 86: 103.

Hörmann G, Lemtis H.: [Defense performances of the "fetus-placenta unit" against the hematogenous transport of cellular combinations of malignant blastomas from the mother]. *Z Geburtshilfe Gynakol.* 1965; 164: 129-42. German.

Hsu HY, Chang MH, Hsieh KH, Lee CY, Lin HH, Hwang LH, Chen PJ, Chen DS.: Cellular immune response to HBcAg in mother-to-infant transmission of hepatitis B virus. *Hepatology* 1992; 15: 770–6.

Hurtado CW, Golden-Mason L, Brocato M, Krull M, Narkewicz MR, Rosen HR.: Innate immune function in placenta and cord blood of hepatitis C-seropositive mother-infant dyads. *PLoS One.* 2010; 5: e12232. DOI: 10.1371/journal.pone.0012232.

Hüser D, Heilbronn R.: Adeno-associated virus integrates site-specifically into human chromosome 19 in either orientation and with equal kinetics and frequency. *J. Gen. Virol.* 2003; 84 (Pt 1): 133-7.

Ikuta K, Ishioka K, Sato Y, Imamura T, Asano K, Koyano S, Inoue N, Suzutania T.: A novel real-time PCR method for determination and quantification of each cytomegalovirus glycoprotein H subtype in clinical samples. *Journal of Clinical Microbiology* 2012; 50: 499–501. DOI:10.1128/JCM.06032-11.

Inchley CS, Sonerud T, Fjærli HO, Nakstad B.: Reduced dicer expression in the cord blood of infants admitted with severe respiratory syncytialvirus disease. *BMC Infect Dis.* 2011; 11: 59-68. DOI:10.1186/1471-2334-11-59.

Ishibashi K, et al. 2007. Association of the outcome of renal transplantation with antibody response to cytomegalovirus strain-specific glycoprotein H epitopes. *Clin. Infect. Dis*. 45:60–67.

Ishibashi K, Yamaguchi O, Suzutani T.: Reinfection of cytomegalovirus in renal transplantation. *Fukushima J. Med. Sci.* 2011; 5: 1-10.

Iso K, Suzuki Y, Takayama M.: Mother-to-infant transmission of TT virus in Japan. *Int. J. Gynaecol Obstet*. 2001; 75: 11-9.

Jacobsen JT, Lunde E, Sundvold-Gjerstad V, Munthe LA, Bogen B.: The cellular mechanism by which complementary Id+ and anti-Id antibodies communicate: T cells integrated into idiotypic regulation. *Immunol Cell Biol.* 2010; 88: 515-22. DOI:10.1038/icb.2009.118.

Jaime-Pérez JC, Colunga-Pedraza JE, Monreal-Robles R, Colunga-Pedraza PR, Méndez-Ramírez N, Salazar-Riojas R, Gómez-Almaguer D.: Acute maternal cytomegalovirus infection is associated with significantly decreased numbers of CD34+ cells in umbilical cord blood. *Blood Cells* Mol Dis. 2012 Jul 17.

Jerne NK.: Towards a network theory of the immune system. *Ann. Immunol.* (Paris). 1974; 125C: 373-89.

Kadereit S, Junge GR, Kleen T, Kozik MM, Kaminski BA, Daum-Woods K, Fu P, Tary-Lehmann M, Laughlin MJ.: Deficient IFN-gamma expression in umbilical cord blood (UCB) T cells can be rescued by IFN-gamma-mediated increase in NFATc2 expression. *J. Clin. Immunol*. 2003; 23: 485-97.

Kékesi Zs, Nika M, Mikola I.: Experiences concerning the hepatitis B screening of pregnant women, and perinatal transmission of the virus [in Hungarian]. *Orvosi Hetilap* 134:1515–20.

Kenneson A, Cannon MJ.: Review and meta-analysis of the epidemiology of congenital cytomegalovirus (CMV) infection. *Revs in Med. Virol* 2007; 17: 253–76.

Kertschanska S, Kosanke G, Kaufman P.: Pressure dependence of so-called transtrophoblastic channels during fetal perfusion of placental villi. *Micros Res Tech* 1997; 38: 52-62. DOI:10.1002/(SICI)1097-0029(19970701/15)38:1/2<52::AID-JEMT7>3.3.CO;2-0.

Kleen T, Kadereit S, Fanning L, Jaroscak J, Fu P, Meyerson HJ, Kulchycki L, Slivka LF, Kozik M, Tary-Lehmann M, Laughlin MJ.: Recipient-specific tolerance after HLA-mismatched umbilical cord blood stem cell transplantation. *Transplantation*. 2005; 9: 1316–22.

Kobayashi D, Kogawa K, Imai K, Tanaka T, Hiroi S, Satoh H, Tanaka-Taya K, Nonoyama S.: Quantitation of human herpesvirus-6 (HHV-6) DNA in a cord blood transplant recipient with chromosomal integration of HHV-6. *Transpl Infect Dis.* 2011; 13: 650-3. DOI: 10.1111/j.1399-3062.2011.00693.x.

Koskimaa HM, Waterboer T, Pawlita M, Grénman S, Syrjänen K, Syrjänen S.: Human papillomavirus genotypes present in the oral mucosa of newborns and their concordance with maternal cervical human papillomavirus genotypes. *J. Pediatr.* 2012; 160: 837-43.

Koumbi LJ, Papadopoulos NG, Anastassiadou V, Machaira M, Kafetzis DA, Papaevangelou V.: Dendritic cells in uninfected infants born to hepatitis B virus-positive mothers. *Clin. Vaccine Immunol.* 2010; 17: 1079-85. DOI: 10.1128/CVI.00074-10.

Kourí V, Correa CB, Verdasquera D, Martínez PA, Alvarez A, Alemán Y, Pérez L, Golpe MA, Someilán T, Chong Y, Fresno C, Navarro MA, Pérez E, Moro I, Sanchez R, Llanusa C, Melin P.: Diagnosis and screening for cytomegalovirus infection in pregnant women in Cuba as prognostic markers of congenital infection in newborns: 2007-2008. *Pediatr. Infect Dis. J.* 2010; 29: 1105-10.

Kovács IJ, Hegedus K, Pál A, Pusztai R.: Production of proinflammatory cytokines by syncytiotrophoblasts infected with human cytomegalovirus isolates. *Placenta* 2007; 28: 620-3.

Krause I, Blank M, Levi Y, Koike T, Barak V, Shoenfeld Y.: Anti-idiotype immunomodulation of experimental anti-phospholipid syndrome via effect on Th1/Th2 expression. *Clin. Exp. Immunol.* 1999; 117: 190-7.

Kwon CI, Hwang SG, Shin SJ, Chang SW, Kim SY, Ko KH, Hong SP, Park PW, Rim KS, Kang MS, Chung HJ, Hong SP.: Occult hepatitis B virus infection in pregnant woman and its clinical implication. *Liver Int.* 2008; 28: 667-74.

Lanier AP, Henle W, Bender TR, Henle G, Talbot ML.: Epstein-Barr virus-specific antibody titers in seven Alaskan natives before and after diagnosis ofnasopharyngeal carcinoma. *Int. J. Cancer.* 1980; 26: 133-7.

Lanier AP, Bulkow LR, Ireland B.: *Cancer in Alaskan Indians, Eskimos, and Aleuts,* 1969-83: implications for etiology and control. Public Health Rep. 1989; 104: 658-64.

Lanier LL, Chang C, Phillips JH.: Human NKR-P1A. A disulfide-linked homodimer of the C-type lectin superfamily expressed by a subset of NK and T lymphocytes. *J. Immunol* 1994; 153: 2417–28.

Law HK, Cheung CY, Sia SF, Chan YO, Peiris JS, Lau YL.: Toll-like receptors, chemokine receptors and death receptor ligands responses in

SARScoronavirus infected human monocyte derived dendritic cells. *BMC Immunol.* 2009;10: 35.

Lemke H, Lange H and Berek C.: Maternal immunization modulates the primary immune response to 2-phenyl-oxazolone in BALB/c mice. *Eur. J. Immunol.* 1994; 24: 3025-30. DOI:10.1002/eji.1830241216.

Lemke H and Lange H.: Is there a maternally induced immunological imprinting phase à la Konrad Lorenz? *Scand J. Immunol.* 1999; 50: 348-54. DOI:10.1046/j.1365-3083.1999.00620.x

Lemke H and Lange H.: Generalization of single immunological experiences by idiotypically mediated clonal connections. *Adv. Immunol.* 2002; 80: 203-41. DOI:10.1016/S0065-2776(02)80016-5.

Lemke H, Coutinho A and Lange H.: Lamarckian inheritance by somatically acquired maternal IgG phenotypes. *Trends Immunol.* 2004; 25: 180-6. doi:10.1016/j.it.2004.02.007.

Lemke H, Tanasa RI, Trad A, Lange H.: Benefits and burden of the maternally-mediated immunological imprinting. *Autoimmun Rev.* 2009; 8: 394-9. doi:10.1016/j.autrev. 2008.12.005.

Lemke H, Tanasa RI, Trad A, Lange H.: Function of maternal idiotypic and anti-idiotypic antibodies as transgenerational messengers. pp 249-80. (Ed. Berencsi G III.) Springer, 2012 . DOI: 10.1007/978-94-007-4216-1_4.

Lenglet Y , Barau G , Robillard PY , Randrianaivo H , Michault A , Bouveret A , Gerardin P , Boumahni B , Touret Y , Kauffmann E , Schuffenecker I , Gabriele M , Fourmaintraux A.: Chikungunya infection in pregnancy: evidence for intrauterine infection in pregnant women and vertical transmission in the parturient. Survey of the Reunion Island outbreak. *J. Gynecol Obstet Biol. Reprod (Paris)* 2006; 35: 578 – 583.

Leruez-Ville M, Vauloup-Fellous C, Couderc S, Parat S, Ouchérif S, Castel C, Magny JF.: [Retrospective diagnosis of congenital CMV infection in DBS from Guthrie cards: French experience]. *Arch. Pediatr.* 2009; 16: 1503-6.

Lin SJ, Cheng PJ, Lin TY, Lee PT, Hsiao HS, Kuo ML.: Effect of influenza A infection on umbilical cord blood natural killer function regulation with interleukin-15. *J. Infect Dis.* 2012; 205: 745-56.

Liu WJ, Huang MX, Guo QL, Chen JH, Shi H.: Effect of human cytomegalovirus infection on the expression of Hoxb2 and Hoxb4 genes in the developmental process of cord blood erythroid progenitors. *Mol. Med. Report.* 2011; 4: 1307-11. DOI: 10.3892/mmr.2011.576.

López M, Coll O.: Chronic viral infections and invasive procedures: risk of vertical transmission and current recommendations. *Fetal Diagn Ther.* 2010; 28: 1-8.

Macdonald N.: Transfusion and risk of infection in Canada: update 2005. *Can. J. Infect Dis. Med. Microbiol* 2005; 16: 161-5.

Maidji E, McDonagh S, Genbacev O, Tabata T, Pereira L.: Maternal antibodies enhance or prevent cytomegalovirus infection in the placenta by neonatal Fc receptor-mediated transcytosis. *Am. J. Pathol* 2006; 168: 1210–26.

Maidji E, Genbacev O, Chang HT, Pereira L.: Developmental regulation of human cytomegalovirus receptors in cytotrophoblasts correlates with distinct replication sites in the placenta. *J. Virol.* 2007; 81: 4701–12.

Maidji E, Nigro G, Tabata T, McDonagh S, Nozawa N, Shiboski S, Muci S, Anceschi MM, Aziz N, Adler SP, Pereira L.: Antibody treatment promotes compensation for human cytomegalovirus-induced pathogenesis and a hypoxia-like condition in placentas with congenital infection. *Am. J. Pathol.* 2010; 177: 1298-310. doi:10.2353/ajpath.2010.091210.

Mannucci S, Luzzi A, Carugi A, Gozzetti A, Lazzi S, Malagnino V, Simmonds M, Cusi MG, Leoncini L, van den Bosch CA, De Falco G.: EBV reactivation and chromosomal polysomies: Euphorbia tirucalli as a possible cofactor in endemic Burkitt Lymphoma. *Adv. Hematol.* 2012; 2012: 149780.

Martin-Latil S, Gnädig NF, Mallet A, Desdouits M, Guivel-Benhassine F, Jeannin P, Prevost MC, Schwartz O, Gessain A, Ozden S, Ceccaldi PE.: Transcytosis of HTLV-1 across a tight human epithelial barrier and infection of subepithelial dendritic cells. *Blood.* 2012; 120: 572-80.

Martinez C, Bragado R, de la Hera A, Toribio ML, Marcos MA, Bandeira A, Pereira P and Coutinho A.: Functional and biochemical evidence for the recognition of T cell receptors by monoclonal antibodies to an immunoglobulin idiotype. *J. Mol. Cell Immunol.* 1986a; 2: 307-13.

Martinez C, Toribio ML, de la Hera A, Cazenave PA and Coutinho A.: Maternal transmission of idiotypic network interactions selecting available T cell repertoires. *Eur. J. Immunol.* 1986b; 16: 1445-7.

Matsubara H, Michitaka K, Horiike N, Kihana T, Yano M, Mori T, Onji M.: Existence of TT virus DNA and TTV-like mini virus DNA in infant cord blood: mother-to-neonatal transmission. *Hepatol. Res.* 2001; 21: 280-7.

Matsuda H, Sakaguchi K, Shibasaki T, Takahashi H, Kawakami Y, Furuya K.: Intrauterine therapy for parvovirus B19 infected symptomatic fetus using B19 IgG-rich high titer gammaglobulin. *J. Perinat. Med.* 2005; 33: 561–3.

Matys K, Mallary S, Bautista O, Vuocolo S, Manalastas R, Pitisuttithum P, Saah A.: Mother-infant transfer of anti-humanpapillomavirus (HPV) antibodies following vaccination with the quadrivalent HPV (type

6/11/16/18) virus-like particle vaccine. *Clin. Vaccine Immunol.* 2012; 19: 881-5.

McIntyre JA.: Immune recognition at the maternal-fetal interface: overview. *Am. J. Reprod. Immunol.* 1992; 28: 127-31. Review.

McLean LK, Chehab FF, Goldberg JD.: Detection of viral deoxyribonucleic acid in the amniotic fluid of low-risk pregnancies by polymerase chain reaction. *Am. J. Obstet Gynecol* 1995; 173: 1282–6.

Miller MA, Weibel C, Kahn JS, Andiman WA.: Seroepidemiology of WU polyomavirus among children exposed perinatally to HIV-1. *J. Med. Virol.* 2012; 84: 188-93. DOI: 10.1002/jmv.23189. 27,4% IgM positivity between 0-5 months of age.

Mix E, Goertsches R, Zett UK.: Immunoglobulins--basic considerations. *J. Neurol.* 2006; 253 Suppl 5:V9-17.

Mouzaki A, Panagoulias I, Raptis G, Farri-Kostopoulou E.: Cord blood leptin levels of healthy neonates are associated with IFN-γ production by cord blood T-cells. *PLoS One*. 2012; 7(7): e40830.

Mrozek-Budzyn D, Kiełtyka A, Majewska R.: Lack of association between measles-mumps-rubella vaccination and autism in children: a case-control study. *Pediatr. Infect. Dis. J.* 2010; 29: 397-400.

Nagamori T, Koyano S, Inoue N, Yamada H, Oshima M, Minematsu T, Fujieda K.: Single cytomegalovirus strain associated with fetal loss and then congenital infection of a subsequent child born to the same mother. *J. Clin. Virol.* 2010; 49: 134-6.

Nakamura T.: HTLV-I-associated myelopathy/tropical spastic paraparesis (HAM/TSP): the role of HTLV-I-infected Th1 cells in the pathogenesis, and therapeutic strategy. *Folia Neuropathol.* 2009;47(2):182-94. Review.

Nasiri R, Yoseffi J, Khajedaloe M, Sarafraz Yazdi M, Delgoshaei F.: Congenital rubella syndrome after rubella vaccination in 1-4 weeks periconceptional period. *Indian J. Pediatr.* 2009; 76: 279-82.

Nishimura M, Sakai K, Akaza T, Mitomi Y, Nieda M, Minami M, Juji T.: Anti-idiotypic antibody to T-cell receptor in multiply transfused patients may play a role in resistance to graft-versus-host disease. *Transfusion.* 1992; 32: 719-28.

Nishishita N, Shikamura M, Takenaka C, Takada N, Fusak N, et al. Generation of virus-free induced pluripotent stem cell clones on a synthetic matrix via a single cell subcloning in the Naı¨ve State. *PLoS ONE* 2012; 7(6): e38389. doi:10.1371/journal.pone.0038389.

Northfield JW, Kasprowicz V, Lucas M, Kersting N, Bengsch B, Kim A, Phillips RE, Walker BD, Thimme R, Lauer G, Klenerman P.: CD161 expression on hepatitis C virus-specific CD8+ T cells suggests a distinct pathway of T cell differentiation. *Hepatology* 2008; 47: 396–406.

Nozawa N, Fang-Hoover J, Tabata T, Maidji E, Pereira L.: Cytomegalovirus-specific, high-avidity IgG with neutralizing activity in maternal circulation enriched in the fetal bloodstream. *J. Clin. Virol.* 2009; 46 Suppl 4: S58-63.

Ohto H, Ujiie N, Sato A, Okamoto H, Mayumi M.: Mother-to-infant transmission of GB virus type C/HGV. *Transfusion.* 2000; 40: 725-30. doi:10.1046/j.1537-2995.2000.40060725.x

Ördög K, Szendrői A, Szarka K, Kugler Z, Csire M, Kapusinszky B, Xie J, Csizmadia K, Brojnás J, Rusvai E, Tempfli A, Berencsi G.: Perinatal and intrafamily transmission of hepatitis b virus in three generations of a low-prevalence population. *J. Med. Virol.* 2003; 70: 194-204. DOI:10.1002/jmv.10378.

Oshimi K, Oshimi Y, Yamada O, Wada M, Hara T, Mizoguchi H.: Cytotoxic T lymphocyte triggering via CD16 is regulated by CD3 and CD8 antigens. Studies with T cell receptor (TCR)-alpha beta+/CD3+16+ and TCR-gamma delta+/CD3+16+ granular lymphocytes. *J. Immunol.* 1990; 144: 3312-7.

Park B, Spooner E, Houser BL, Strominger JL, Ploegh HL.: The HCMV membrane glycoprotein US10 selectively targets HLA-G for degradation. *JEM* 2010; 207: 2033-41.

Peckham CS.: Cytomegalovirus infection: congenital and neonatal disease. *Scand J. Infect Dis.* 1991; 80: 82–7.

Peigo MF, Thomasini RL, Puglia AL, Costa SC, Bonon SH, Boin IF, Leonardi M, Mota NG.: Human herpesvirus-7 in Brazilian liver transplant recipients: a follow-up comparison between molecular and immunological assays. *Transpl Infect Dis.* 2009; 11: 497-502.

Peled Y, Yogev Y, Oron G, Amir J, Pardo J.: Suggested algorithm for cytomegalovirus surveillance in low-risk pregnancies. *J. Matern Fetal Neonatal Med.* 2011; 24: 1353-6.

Pellett PE, Ablashi DV, Ambros PF, Agut H, Caserta MT, Descamps V, Flamand L, Gautheret-Dejean A, Hall CB, Kamble RT, Kuehl U, Lassner D, Lautenschlager I, Loomis KS, Luppi M, Lusso P, Medveczky PG, Montoya JG, Mori Y, Ogata M, Pritchett JC, Rogez S, Seto E, Ward KN, Yoshikawa T, Razonable RR.: Chromosomally integrated human herpesvirus 6: questions and answers. *Rev. Med. Virol.* 2012; 22: 144-55. DOI: 10.1002/rmv.715.

Pereira L, Maidji E, Fisher SJ, McDonagh S, Tabata T.: HCMV persistence in the population: potential transplacental transmission. In: Arvin A,

Campadelli-Fiume G, Mocarski E, Moore PS, Roizman B, Whitley R, Yamanishi K, editors. Human Herpesviruses: *Biology, Therapy, and Immunoprophylaxis*. Cambridge: Cambridge University Press; 2007. Chapter 45.

Pessina A, Bonomi A, Coccè V, Bernardo ME, Cometa AM, Ferrari M, Sisto F, Cavicchini L, Locatelli F.: Assessment of human herpesvirus-6 infection in mesenchymal stromal cells ex vivo expanded for clinical use. *Transpl Infect Dis*. 2009; 11: 491-6.

Petrikovsky BM, Lipson SM, Kaplan MH.: Viral studies on amniotic fluid from fetuses with and without abnormalities detected by prenatal sonography. *J. Reprod. Med.* 2003; 48: 230–232.

Pichereau C, Desseaux K, Janin A, Scieux C, Peffault de Latour R, Xhaard A, Robin M, Ribaud P, Agbalika F, Chevret S, Socié G.: The complex relationship between human herpesvirus 6 and acute graft-versus-host disease. *Biol. Blood Marrow Transplant*. 2012; 18: 141-4.

Pinon JM, Dumon H, Chemla C, Franck J, Petersen E, Lebech M, Zufferey J, Bessieres MH, Marty P, Holliman R, Johnson J, Luyasu V, Lecolier B, Guy E, Joynson DH, Decoster A, Enders G, Pelloux H, Candolfi E .: Strategy for diagnosis of congenital toxoplasmosis: evaluation of methods comparing mothers and newborns and standard methods for postnatal detection of immunoglobulin G, M, and A antibodies. *J. Clin. Microbiol* 2001; 39: 2267-71.

Plans P, Costa J, Domínguez A, Torner N, Borras E, Plasència A.: Prevalence of protective measles virus antibody levels in umbilical cord blood samples in Catalonia, Spain. *Clin. Vaccine Immunol.* 2010; 17: 691-4.

Pol S, Corouge M, Fontaine H.: Hepatitis B virus infection and pregnancy. *Clin. Res. Hepatol. Gastroenterol.* 2011; 35: 618-22.

Prabakaran P, Zhu Z, Chen W, Gong R, Feng Y, Streaker E, Dimitrov DS.: Origin, diversity, and maturation of human antiviral antibodies analyzed by high-throughput sequencing. *Front Microbiol.* 2012; 3: 277.

Prabakaran P, Chen W, Singarayan MG, Stewart CC, Streaker E, Feng Y, Dimitrov DS.: Expressed antibody repertoires in human cord blood cells: 454 sequencing and IMGT/HighV-QUEST analysis of germline gene usage, junctional diversity, and somatic mutations. *Immunogenetics.* 2012; 64: 337-50.

Pradhan M, Anand B, Singh A.: Hepatitis E Virus Infection Causing Isolated Fetal Ascites: A Case Report. *Fetal Diagn Ther.* 2012 Jun 1. DOI: 10.1159/000337612

Qin J, Goswami R, Balabanov R, Dawson G.: Oxidized phosphatidylcholine is a marker for neuroinflammation in multiple sclerosis brain. *J. Neurosci Res.* 2007; 85: 977-84.

Randolph-Habecker J, Iwata M, Torok-Storb B.: Cytomegalovirus mediated myelosuppression. *J. Clin. Virol.* 2002; 25 (Suppl. 2) S51–S56.

Rastogi D, Wang C, Mao X, Lendor C, Rothman PB, Miller RL.: Antigen-specific immune responses to influenza vaccine in utero. *J. Clin. Invest.* 2007; 117: 1637-46.

Reddy UM, Baschat AA, Zlatnik MG, Towbin JA, Harman CR, Weiner CP. Detection of viral deoxyribonucleic acid in amniotic fluid: association with fetal malformation and pregnancy abnormalities. *Fetal Diagn Ther* 2005; 20: 203–207.

Redman CW, Sargent IL.: Circulating microparticles in normal pregnancy and pre-eclampsia. Placenta 2008; 29 Suppl A: S73-7. DOI:10.1016/j.placenta.2007.11.016

Renneson J, Dutta B, Goriely S, Danis B, Lecomte S, Laes JF, Tabi Z, Goldman M, Marchant A.: IL-12 and type I IFN response of neonatal myeloid DC to human CMV infection. *Eur. J. Immunol.* 2009; 39: 2789-99.

Rice PS, Cason J, Best JM, Banatvala JE.: High risk genital papillomavirus infections are spread vertically. *Rev. Med. Virol.* 1999; 9: 15–21.

Rice PS, Mant C, Cason J, Bible JM, Muir P, Kell B, Best JM.: High prevalence of human papillomavirus type 16 infection among children. *J. Med. Virol.* 2000; 61: 70–75.

Romano L, Paladini S, Van Damme P, Zanetti AR.: The worldwide impact of vaccination on the control and protection of viral hepatitis b. *Dig. Liver Dis* 2011; 43 Suppl 1: S2-7. DOI:10.1016/S1590-8658(10)60685-8.

Roth DE, Jones AB, Prosser C, Robinson JL, Vohra S.: Vitamin D receptor polymorphisms and the risk of acute lower respiratory tract infection in early childhood. *J. Infect Dis.* 2008; 197: 676 – 80.

Rölle A, Olweus J.: Dendritic cells in CMV infection: viral evasion and host countermeasures. *APMIS* 2009; 117: 413–26.

Rudensky AY, Mazel SM, Blechman JM and Yurin VL.: Immunoglobulin-specific T-B cell interaction. IV. B cell presentation of idiotypic determinant(s) of monoclonal anti-surface immunoglobulin antibody to idiotope-recognizing helper T clones. *Eur. J. Immunol.* 1990; 20: 1691-6. DOI:10.1002/eji.1830200811.

Rugolotto S, Padovani EM, Sanna A, Chiaffoni GP, Marradi PL, Borgna-Pignatti C.: Intrauterine anemia due to parvovirus B19: successful treatment with intravenous immunoglobulins. *Haematologica* 1999; 84: 668–9.

Sadeghi M, Riipinen A, Väisänen E, Chen T, Kantola K, Surcel HM, Karikoski R, Taskinen H, Söderlund-Venermo M, Hedman K.: Newly discovered KI, WU, and Merkel cell polyomaviruses: no evidence of mother-to-fetus transmission. *Virol J.* 2010; 7: 251. DOI:10.1186/1743-422X-7-251.

Sadeghian MH, Katebi M, Ayatollahi H, Keramati MR.: Immunohistochemical study association between human herpesvirus 8 and multiple myeloma. *Int. J. Hematol.* 2008; 88: 283-6.

Samson M, Jung D.: Intracellular trafficking and fate of chimeric adenovirus 5/F35 in human B lymphocytes. *J. Gene Med.* 2011; 13: 451-61. doi: 10.1002/jgm.1588.

Sanchez MA, Bello-Munoz JC, Cebrecos I, Sanz TH, Martinez JS, Moratonas EC, Roura LC.: The prevalence of congenital varicella syndrome after a maternal infection, but before 20 weeks of pregnancy: a prospective cohort study. *J. Matern Fetal Neonatal. Med.* 2011; 24: 341-7.

Sarkola ME, Grénman SE, Rintala MA, Syrjänen KJ, Syrjänen SM.: Human papillomavirus in the placenta and umbilical cord blood. *Acta Obstet Gynecol Scand.* 2008; 87: 1181-8.

Sarfraz AA, Samuelsen SO, Bruu AL, Jenum PA, Eskild A.: Maternal human parvovirus B19 infection and the risk of fetal death and low birthweight: a case-control study within 35 940 pregnant women. *BJOG.* 2009; 116: 1492-8.

Schaefer O, Hildes JA, Medd LM, Cameron DG.: The changing pattern of neoplastic disease in Canadian Eskimos. *Can. Med. Assoc J.* 1975;112:1399-404.

Schweintzger S, Schlagenhauf A, Leschnik B, Rinner B, Bernhard H, Novak M, Muntean W.: Microparticles in newborn cord blood: slight elevation after normal delivery. *Thromb Res.* 2011; 128: 62-7.

Selbing A, Josefsson A, Dahle LO, Lindgren R.: Parvovirus B19 infection during pregnancy treated with high-dose intravenous gammaglobulin. *Lancet* 1995; 345:660–1.

Setiady YY, Samy ET and Tung KS.: Maternal autoantibody triggers de novo T cell-mediated neonatal autoimmune disease. *J. Immunol.* 2003; 170: 4656-64.

Shi Z, Yang Y, Wang H, Ma L, Schreiber A, Li X, Sun W, Zhao X, Yang X, Zhang L, Lu W, Teng J, An Y.: Breastfeeding of newborns by mothers carrying hepatitis B virus: a meta-analysis and systematic review. *Arch Pediatr. Adolesc. Med.* 2011; 165: 837-46.

Simmons P, Kaushansky K, Torok-Storb B.: Mechanisms of cytomegalovirus-mediated myelosuppression: perturbation of stromal cell function versus direct infection of myeloid cells, *Proc. Natl. Acad. Sci. USA*. 1990; 87: 1386–90.

Sinkovics JG.: Antileukemia and antitumor effects of the graft-versus-host disease: a new immunovirological approach. *Acta Microbiol Immunol Hung*. 2010; 57: 253-347. Review.

Sloma I, Imren S, Beer PA, Zhao Y, Lecault V, Leung D, Raghuram K, Brimacombe C, Lambie K, Piret J, Hansen C, Humphries RK, Eaves CJ.: Ex vivo expansion of normal and chronic myeloid leukemic stem cells without functional alteration using a NUP98HOXA10 homeodomain fusion gene. *Leukemia*. 2012 Jul 16. doi: 10.1038/leu.2012.196.

Smith-Norowitz TA, Norowitz KB, Silverberg JI, Chice S, Shah V, Stanek A, Walker D, Brennan JP, Durkin HG, Bluth MH.: CD8+CD60+ T cells, cells expressing epsilon specific mRNA and Th1/Th2 cytokines in cord blood and at 7 months of age. *Scand. J. Immunol*. 2008; 68: 526-33.

Solves P, Mirabet V, Alvarez M, Vila E, Quiles F, Villalba JV, Montoro JA, Soler MA, Roig RJ.: Donor screening for hepatitis B virus infection in a cell and tissue bank. *Transpl. Infect Dis*. 2008; 10: 391-5.

Srivatsa B, Srivatsa S, Johnson KL, Samura O, Lee SL, Bianchi DW.: Microchimerism of presumed fetal origin in thyroid specimens from women: a case-control study. *Lancet* 2001; 358: 2034–8. doi:10.1016/S0140-6736(01)07099-4.

Srivatsa B, Srivatsa S, Johnson KL, Bianchi DW.: Maternal cell microchimerism in newborn tissues. *J. Pediatr.* 2003; 142: 31-5. doi:10.1067/mpd.2003.mpd0327.

Stagno S, Reynolds DW, Huang ES, Thames SD, Smith RJ, Alford CA: Congenital cytomegalovirus infection. *N Engl. J. Med*. 1977: 296: 1254–8.

Stea EA, Routsias JG, Clancy RM, Buyon JP, Moutsopoulos HM and Tzioufas AG.: Anti-La/SSB antiidiotypic antibodies in maternal serum: a marker of low risk for neonatal lupus in an offspring. *Arthritis Rheum*. 2006; 54: 2228-34. DOI:10.1002/art.21954.

Steiner, K., Myrie, L., Malhotra, I., Mungai, P., Muchiri, E., Dent, A., King, C.L., 2010. Fetal immune activation to malaria antigens enhances susceptibility to in vitro HIV infection in cord blood mononuclear cells. *J. Infect. Dis*. 202 (6), 899–907.

Steiner KL, Malhotra I, Mungai PL, Muchiri EM, Dent AE, King CL.: In utero activation of fetal memory T cells alters host regulatory gene expression and affects HIV susceptibility. *Virology.* 2012; 425: 23-30.

Stern M, Ruggeri L, Mancusi A, Bernardo ME, de Angelis C, Bucher C, Locatelli F, Aversa F, Velardi A.:Survival after T cell-depleted haploidentical stem cell transplantation is improved using the mother as donor. *Blood* 2008; 112: 2990–5. doi:10.1182/blood-2008-01-135285.

Stinson K, Boulle A, Smith PJ, Stringer EM, Stringer JS, Coetzee D.: Coverage of the prevention of mother-to-child transmission program in the Western Cape, South Africa using cord blood surveillance. *J. Acquir Immune Defic Syndr.* 2012; 60: 199-204. DOI: 10.1097/QAI. 0b013e31824d985e.

Straub I.: Experiences of the introduction of country-wide programme for the prevention of hepatitis B virus infection of newborns [in Hungarian]. Epinfo 1996; 3: 225–232.

Strong DM, Katz L.: Blood-bank testing for infectious diseases: how safe is blood transfusion? *Trends Mol. Med* 2002; 8: 355-8.

Sullivan BM, Coscoy L.: Downregulation of the T-cell receptor complex and impairment of T-cell activation by human herpesvirus 6 U24 protein. *J. Virol.* 2008; 82: 602–608.

Sumino K, Tucker J, Shahab M, Jaffee KF, Visness CM, Gern JE, Bloomberg GR, Holtzman MJ.: Antiviral IFN-γ responses of monocytes at birth predict respiratory tract illness in the first year of life. *J. Allergy Clin. Immunol.* 2012; 129: 1267-73.e1.

Sundaravaradan V, Mehta R, Harris DT, Zack JA, Ahmad N.: Differential expression and interaction of host factors augment HIV-1 gene expression in neonatal mononuclear cells. *Virology* 2010; 400: 32–43.

Sur DK, Wallis DH, O'Connell TX.: Vaccinations in pregnancy. *Am. Fam. Physician.* 2003; 68: 299-304.

Svensson A, Nordström I, Rudin A, Bergström T, Eriksson K.: Enveloped virus but not bacteria block IL-13 responses in human cord blood T cells in vitro. *Scand. J. Immunol.* 2012; 75: 409-18. doi: 10.1111/j.1365-3083.2012.02676.x.

Syrjänen S.: Current concepts on human papillomavirus infections in children. *APMIS.* 2010; 118) :494-509. Review.

Szabolcs P, Niedzwiecki D.: Immune reconstitution after unrelated cord blood transplantation. *Cytotherapy.* 2007; 9: 111–122.

Szabolcs P, Cairo MS.: Unrelated umbilical cord blood transplantation and immune reconstitution. *Semin. Hematol.* 2010; 47: 22-36. Review

Széles L, Keresztes G, Töröcsik D, Balajthy Z, Krenács L, Póliska S, Steinmeyer A, Zuegel U, Pruenster M, Rot A, Nagy L.: 1,25-Dihydroxyvitamin D3 is an autonomous regulator of the transcriptional changes leading to a tolerogenic dendritic cell phenotype. *J. Immunol.* 2009; 182: 2074 –83.

Tagawa M, Tanaka H, Moriuchi M, Moriuchi H.: Retrospective diagnosis of congenital cytomegalovirus infection at a school for the deaf by using preserved dried umbilical cord. *J. Pediatr.* 2009; 155: 749-51.

Takahashi T, Ozawa K, Takahashi K, Asano S, Takaku F.: Susceptibility of human erythropoietic cells to B19 parvovirus in vitro increases with differentiation. *Blood* 1990; 75: 603–610.

Tan PC, Rajasingam G, Devi S, Omar SZ.: Dengue infection in pregnancy: prevalence, vertical transmission, and pregnancy outcome. *Obstet Gynecol.* 2008; 111: 1111-7.

Tan PT, Heiny AT, Miotto O, Salmon J, Marques ET, Lemonnier F, August JT.: Conservation and diversity of influenza A H1N1 HLA-restricted T cell epitope candidates for epitope-based vaccines. *PLoS One.* 2010 Jan 18;5(1):e8754.

Tanaka-Taya K, Sashihara J, Kurahashi H, Amo K, Miyagawa H, Kondo K, Okada S, Yamanishi K.: Human herpesvirus 6 (HHV-6) is transmitted from parent to child in an integrated form and characterization of cases with chromosomally integrated HHV-6 DNA. *J. Med. Virol.* 2004; 73: 465–73.

Tanasa RI, Trad A, Lange H, Grötzinger J and Lemke H.: Allergen IgE-isotype-specific suppression by maternally derived monoclonal anti-IgG-idiotype. *Allergy.* 2010; 65: 16-23. DOI:10.1111/j.1398-9995.2009.02104.x.

Theiler RN, Caliendo AM, Pargman S, Raynor BD, Berga S, McPheeters M, Jamieson DJ.: Umbilical cord blood screening for cytomegalovirus DNA by quantitative PCR. *J. Clin. Virol.* 2006; 37: 313-6.

Touret Y , Randrianaivo H , Michault A , Schuffenecker I , Kauffmann E , Lenglet Y , Barau G , Fourmaintraux A.: Early maternal-fetal transmission of the Chikungunya virus . *Presse Med.* 2006; 35: 1656 – 8 .

Toyoda H, Naruse M, Yokozaki S, Morita K, Nakano I, Itakura A, Okamura M, Fukuda Y, Hayakawa T.: Prevalence of infection with TT virus (TTV), a novel DNA virus, in healthy Japanese subjects, newborn infants, cord blood and breast milk. *J. Infect.* 1999; 38: 198-9. doi:10.1016/S0163-4453(99)90254-2.

Traiber C, Coelho-Amaral P, Ritter VR, Winge A.: Infant meningoencephalitis caused by yellow fever vaccine virus transmitted via breastmilk. *J. Pediatr.* (Rio J) 2011; 87: 269-72.

Trlifajová J, Benda R, Benes C.: Effect of maternal varicella-zoster virus infection on the outcome of pregnancy and the analysis of transplacental virus transmission. *Acta Virol.* 1986; 30: 249-55.

Trottier H, Buteau C, Robitaille N, Duval M, Tucci M, Lacroix J, Alfieri C.: Transfusion-related Epstein-Barr virus infection among stem cell transplant recipients: a retrospective cohort study in children. *Transfusion.* 2012; doi: 10.1111/j.1537-2995.2012.03611.x.

Tsatsaris V, Capitant C, Schmitz T, Chazallon C, Bulifon S, Riethmuller D, Picone O, Poulain P, Lewin F, Lainé F, Jacqz-Aigrain E, Aboulker JP, Launay O, Inserm C09-33, PREFLUVAC (Immunogenicity and Safety of an Inactivated Nonadjuvanted A[H1N1v] Influenza Vaccine in Pregnant Women) Study Group.: Maternal immune response and neonatal seroprotection from a single dose of a monovalent nonadjuvanted 2009 influenza A(H1N1) vaccine: a single-group trial. *Ann. Intern. Med.* 2011; 155: 733-41.

Tseng YR, Wu JF, Ni YH, Chen HL, Chen CC, Wen WH, Hsu HY, Chang MH.: Long-term effect of maternal HBeAg on delayed HBeAg seroconversion in offspring with chronic hepatitis B infection. *Liver Int.* 2011 Oct;31(9):1373-80. doi: 10.1111/j.1478-3231.2011.02574.x.

Vaheri A, Vesikari T, Oker-Blom N, Seppala M, Veronelli J, Robbins FC, Parkman PD.: Transmission of attenuated rubella vaccines to the human fetus. A preliminary report. *Am. J. Dis. Child.* 1969; 118: 243-6.

Vaheri A, Vesikari T, Oker-Blom N, Seppala M, Parkman PD, Veronelli J, Robbins FC.: Isolation of attenuated rubella-vaccine virus from human products of conception and uterine cervix. *N Engl. J. Med.* 1972; 286: 1071-4.

Vallhov H, Gutzeit C, Johansson SM, Nagy N, Paul M, Li Q, Friend S, George TC, Klein E, Scheynius A, Gabrielsson S.: Exosomes containing glycoprotein 350 released by EBV-transformed B cells selectively target B cells through CD21 and block EBV infection in vitro. *J. Immunol.* 2011; 186: 73-82.

Vamvakas EC.: Is human herpesvirus-8 transmitted by transfusion? *Transfus Med. Rev.* 2010; 24: 1-14.

Van den Veyver IB, Ni J, Bowles N, Carpenter RJ Jr, Weiner CP, Yankowitz J, Moise KJ Jr, Henderson J, Towbin JA.: Detection of intrauterine viral infection using the polymerase chain reaction. *Mol. Genet Metab.* 1998; 63: 85–95.

van Halteren AG, Jankowska-Gan E, Joosten A, Blokland E, Pool J, Brand A, Burlingham WJ, Goulmy E.: Naturally acquired tolerance and sensitization to minor histocompatibility antigens in healthy family members. *Blood.* 2009; 114: 2263-72. doi:10.1182/blood-2009-01-200410.

van Rood JJ, Scaradavou A, Stevens CE.: Indirect evidence that maternal microchimerism in cord blood mediates a graft-versus-leukemia effect in cord bloodtransplantation. *Proc. Natl. Acad. Sci. USA*. 2012; 109: 2509–14. doi: 10.1073/pnas.1119541109.

Vermijlen D, Brouwer M, Donner C, Liesnard C, Tackoen M, Van Rysselberge M, Twité N, Goldman M, Marchant A, Willems F.: Human cytomegalovirus elicits fetal gammadelta T cell responses in utero. *J. Exp Med.* 2010; 207:807-21.

Walker CM, van Burik JA, De For TE, Weisdorf DJ.: Cytomegalovirus infection after allogeneic transplantation: comparison of cord blood with peripheral blood and marrow graft sources. *Biol. Blood Marrow Transplant.* 2007; 13: 1106–15.

Wang Q, Liu H, Zhang X, Liu Q, Xing Y, Zhou X, Tong C, Zhu P.: High doses of mother's lymphocyte infusion to treat EBV-positive T-cell lymphoproliferative disorders in childhood. *Blood.* 2010; 116: 5941-7.

Warrington RJ, Wong SK, Ramdahin S, Rutherford WJ.: Normal human cord blood B cells can produce high affinity IgG antibodies to dsDNA that are recognized by cord blood-derived anti-idiotypic antibodies. *Scand J. Immunol.* 1995; 42: 397–406.

Watanabe T, Kawamura T, Jacob SE, Aquilino EA, Orenstein JM, Black JB, Blauvelt A.: Pityriasis rosea is associated with systemic active infection with both human herpesvirus-7 and human herpesvirus-6. *J. Invest Dermatol.* 2002; 119: 793–7.

Weiffenbach J, Bald R, Gloning KP, Minderer S, Gärtner BC, Weidner A, Hanke M, Enders M.: Serological and virological analysis of maternal and fetal blood samples in prenatal human parvovirus b19 infection. *J. Infect Dis.* 2012; 205: 782-8.

Wenstrom KD, Andrews WW, Bowles NE, Towbin JA, Hauth JC, Goldenberg RL.: Intrauterine viral infection at the time of second trimester genetic amniocentesis. *Obstet. Gynecol.* 1998; 92: 420–4.

Wernet P, Trapp T, Zweigerdt R, Mann J, Trompeter HI.: Lentiviral labeling reveals three germ layer differentiation potential of a single unrestricted somatic stem cell from human cord blood. *Exp. Hematol.* 2010; 38: 1099-104. doi: 10.1016/j.exphem.2010.09.006.

World Health Organization. Antiretroviral Drugs for Treating Pregnant Women and Preventing HIV Infection in Infants: Recommendations for a Public Health Approach. Geneva, Switzerland: World Health Organization; 2010.

Wu JF, Chen CH, Hsieh RP, Shih HH, Chen YH, Li CR, Chiang CY, Shau WY, Ni YH, Chen HL, Hsu HY, Chang MH.: HLA typing associated with hepatitis B E antigen seroconversionin children with chronic hepatitis B virus infection: a long-term prospective sibling cohort study in Taiwan. *J. Pediatr.* 2006; 148: 647-51

Wu JY, Liao C, Xu ZP, Chen JS, Gu SL, Huang YN, Li Y, Tang XW, Yang X, Tang PH, Tsang KS.: Banking and transplantation of umbilical cord blood in Guangzhou, China, *Cytotherapy* 2006; 8: 488–97.

Wu JF, Ni YH, Lin YT, Lee TJ, Hsu SH, Chen HL, Tsuei DJ, Hsu HY, Chang MH.: Human interleukin-10 genotypes are associated with different precore/core gene mutation patterns in children with chronic hepatitis B virus infection. *J. Pediatr.* 2011; 158: 808-13.

Wu TW, Lin HH, Wang LY.: Chronic hepatitis B infection in adolescents who had received primary infantile vaccination. *Hepatology*. 2012 Aug 1. doi: 10.1002/hep.25988.

Xiao X, Chen W, Feng Y, Zhu Z, Prabakaran P, Wang Y, Zhang MY, Longo NS, Dimitrov DS.: Germline-like predecessors of broadly neutralizing antibodies lack measurable binding to HIV-1 envelope glycoproteins: implications for evasion of immune responses and design of vaccine immunogens. *Biochem. Biophys. Res. Commun.* 2009; 390: 404–409.

Yagami Y.: [Pathogenesis on infertility; its immunological aspects]. Nihon Sanka Fujinka Gakkai Zasshi. 1993; 45: 735-47. [Article in Japanese]

Yogeswaran K, Fung SK.: Chronic hepatitis B in pregnancy: unique challenges and opportunities. *Korean J. Hepatol.* 2011; 17: 1–8. DOI: 10.3350/kjhep.2011.17.1.1.

Yoshida K, Furumoto H, Abe A, Kato T, Nishimura M, Kuwahara A, Maeda K, Matsuzaki T, Irahara M.: The possibility of vertical transmission of human papillomavirus through maternal milk. *J. Obstet. Gynaecol.* 2011; 31: 503-6.

Yoshida M, Matsuda H, Hasegawa Y, Yoshinaga Y, Asai K, Kawashima A, Furuya K.: Accumulation of fetal IgG in immunoglobulin injection into the fetal abdominal cavity is proven. *Fetal Diagn Ther.* 2011; 29: 229-32. doi: 10.1159/000322041.

Yoshida M, Matsuda H, Yoshinaga Y, Asai K, Kawashima A, Sei K, Furuya K.: Can measurement of maternal anti-cytomegalovirus immunoglobulin-M antibody levels be used to screen for cytomegalovirus infection in embryos and fetuses? *J. Obstet Gynaecol. Res*. 2012 Jun 4. doi: 10.1111/j.1447-0756.2012.01900.x.

Yuste RS, Frías C, López A, Vallejo C, Martín P, Bellas C.: Diagnostic value of JC/BK virusantibody immunohistochemistry staining in urine samples from posttransplant immunosuppressed patients in relation to polyomavirus reactivation. *Acta Cytol*. 2008; 52: 191-5.

Younes SA, Csire M, Palyi B, Mikala G, Vályi-Nagy I, Cseh I, Benczik M, Jeney C, Takács T, Simon E, Fülöp V, Berencsi G, Fekete G, Visy M.: Endotoxins do not influence transplacental transmission of lymphotropic human herpesviruses and human papillomaviruses into amniotic fluid taken from healthy mothers before parturition in Hungary. *Acta Microbiol Immunol. Hung*. 2007; 54: 279-303.

Younes Saleh Ali, Csire M, Kapusinszky B, Szomor K, Takács M, Berencsi G.: Heterogeneous Pathways of Maternal-fetal Transmission of Human Viruses (Review). *Pathol. Oncol. Res* 2009; 15: 451–65. DOI 10.1007/s12253-009-9166-9.

Zhao Y, Liu Y, Chen Z, Korteweg C, Gu J.: Immunoglobulin g (IgG) expression in human umbilical cord endothelial cells. *J. Histochem Cytochem*. 2011; 59: 474-88.

Zheng Y, Lu Y, Ye Q, Xia Y, Zhou Y, Yao Q, Wei S.: Should chronic hepatitis B mothers breastfeed? a meta analysis. *BMC Public Health*. 2011; 11: 502-12. DOI:10.1186/1471-2458-11-502.

Zhu YY, Mao YZ, Wu WL, Cai QX, Lin XH.: Does hepatitis B virus prenatal transmission result in postnatal immunoprophylaxis failure? *Clin. Vaccine Immunol*. 2010; 17: 1836-41.

In: Cord Blood
Editor: Lisandra Vanostrand

ISBN: 978-1-62618-072-7

Chapter 2

Mesenchymal Stem Cells and its Role in Regenerative Medicine Applications

Prathibha Shetty*[*]*, Shabari Sarang and Chandra Viswanathan
Regenerative Medicine Group , Reliance life Sciences Pvt Ltd, Dhirubhai Ambani Life Sciences Centre, Rabale, Navi Mumbai

Abstract

Introduction

Current treatments for various degenerative disorders rely on surgical interventions and drugs that modulate the system, but these have their own limitations when it comes to regeneration of damaged tissues and cells. To address this shortcoming, cell-based therapies are gaining importance. Adult stem cells have generated great amount of interest amongst the scientific community for their potential therapeutic applications for unmet medical needs. Haematopoietic stem cells and MSCs are the two widely studied and characterized adult stem cells.

[*] Correspondence: Dr. Prathibha Shetty, Reliance Life Sciences Pvt Ltd, Dhirubhai Ambani Life, Sciences Centre, R-282, TTC Area of MIDC, Thane Belapur Road, Rabale, Navi Mumbai-400701, India Tel. +91.226.767.8436 - Fax: +91.226.767.8099ù, E-mail: prathibha.shetty@ relbio.com.

Mesenchymal stem cells as a choice for cell-based therapies in regenerative medicine are becoming very clear.

Sources for MSCs

Currently, BM represents the main source of MSCs for both experimental and clinical studies, but with limitations. Bone marrow - mesenchymal stem cells have been used in several clinical trials in various domains, such as, cardiology, neurology, and so on, with its limitations in the autologous settings, as it represents 0.01-0.001% of the nucleated cells in the adult human marrow. Hence, to overcome these limitations there is a need for an alternative source, which is easily available, noncontroversial, and could generate a higher number of MSCs. Therefore, the search for alternative sources of MSCs is of significant value. Of these different sources, human umbilical cord blood, cord tissue and adipose tissue could successfully replace BM as a source for MSCs.

Characterization of MSCs

MSCs, as defined by the International Society for Cellular Therapy (ISCT), are multipotent, spindle like plastic adherent cells capable of self-renewal and possess the ability to differentiate *in vitro* to bone, cartilage and adipose tissues. Phenotypic characterization studies of MSCs have shown that these cells express CD73, CD105, CD90, CD29 and CD44 cell surface antigens, and are negative for CD34, CD45, CD31, CD14, human leukocyte antigen (HLA)-class II antigens and von Willebrand factor. Recently some interesting molecules were described which may be useful to identify MSC (sub) populations (CD271, GD2, CD49a, W7C5, W8B2, C15, CDCP1, CD340, CD349, SSEA1/4). However, a distinct exclusively MSC-restricted marker has yet to be identified.

Differentiation to Mesodermal, Ectodermal and Endodermal Lineages

In vitro differentiation studies have shown that MSCs could differentiate to additional cell types encompassing mesodermal (myocytes and tendon), as well as cells of ectodermal (neurons) and endodermal (hepatocytes, pancreatic) lineages. Various studies induced MSC differentiation into neurons and glial cells. After *in vitro* neural differentiation cells demonstrated an assortment of neuronal and glial markers, such as neuronspecific enolase (NSE), neuronal nuclear antigen

(NeuN), neurofilament M (NF-M), tau, glial fibrillary acidic protein (GFAP) and adopted neuronal and glial morphology. Rat MSC were stimulated to differentiate into cells with hepatocyte-like phenotypes after treatment with HGF.

Preclinical Studies

Animal studies have provided a useful tool for defining a number of diverse potential applications for MSCs. Recent studies have shown that BMMSCs improve neurological deficits when transplanted into animal models of neurological disorders. Studies in rodents suggest a broad initial biodistribution followed by a limited capacity for sustained engraftment. In fetal sheep, MSCs undergo a wide tissue distribution and can differentiate into multiple mesenchymal tissues following peritoneal implantation.It has been demonstrated that cultured mesenchymal cells could home to the bone marrow in non-human primates.

Immunological aspects of MSCs

First, the MSCs have the ability to repopulate the damaged host tissue for repair and restoration and second, these cells exert their immunomodulatory and immunosuppressive properties to survive in allogeneic hosts. *In vivo* observations after administration of MSC, like improvement of the outcome after allogeneic transplantations by promotion of hematopoietic engraftment and amelioration of graftversus-host disease as well as the amelioration of inflammatory response and improved clinical course in experimental allergic encephalomyelitis are impressive proofs for the immunomodulatory properties of MSC. Experimental data suggest that both cell surface molecules and soluble factors regulate the hypoimmunogenic, anti-inflammatory and anti-proliferative properties of MSCs

Clinical Applications

In vivo transplantation of undifferentiated MSCs from various tissues, predominantly from the bone marrow, has shown therapeutic efficacy in experimental models of human diseases. All these properties of MSCs, along with their non-tumorigenic nature, have made them attractive candidate for human clinical use, mainly in autologous cell transplantation to treat degenerative diseases. MSCs are currently studied as treatment for inflammatory diseases such as graft-versus host--disease, but also as treatment for myocardial infarct and solid organ transplantation.

Conclusion

MSCs can be differentiated into distinct different skeletal tissues both in *vitro* and *in vivo*. This versatile and tunable differentiation potential of MSCs in conjunction with their ability to secrete various trophic factors and modulate the recipient's immune system makes them a promising cell source in regenerative medicine. Most of the research has been done in the last decade focusing on characterizing MSCs and understanding their differentiation potential. However, the complex mechanisms and pathways with which MSCs supports repair are far from fully understood.Their immunosuppressive capabilities without evidence of immunosuppressive toxicity at a global level define their application in the treatment of diseases in which the pathogenesis involves uncontrolled activity of the immune system.

Introduction

Every century has its own set of significant events, in every sphere of the social setting prevalent then. Some events are significant for a region, some for a nation and a few make a mark in the history of the world. Regenerative medicine sure did make the cut as one of the most significant scientific advances in the recent times. What makes regenerative medicine such an award winning concept is the promise that it holds for every living person, in every part of the world. The Achilles heel is to take this fascinating concept from the laboratory to the bed side. After all the debate over ethics, human rights and legalities, mankind has reached a win some conclusion- "let stem cell therapy enter the markets and may it benefit as many people as is possible." While this magnanimous approach brought a cheer from scientists and regenerative medicine enthusiasts, we have still to fine tune the chinks in the system governing the use of stem cells. We can say that mankind has had enough time to get its act together on regularizing the use of stem cells. After all, it was the Greek Titan, Prometheus, who is said to have experienced the miracles of the regenerative power of the human body- so many centuries ago! The story, as it goes, was this- As punishment for giving fire to Humankind, Zeus ordered Prometheus chained to a rock and sent an eagle to eat his liver each day. However, Prometheus' liver was able to regenerate itself daily, enabling him to survive. It has been a long, arduous journey since then. We have progressed from not being able to deal with this astounding discovery and finally being able to conjure up the courage to test the practical applicability of stem cells.

Our progress from experimental organ transplants, to clinically accepted organ transplants, to the use of medical devices to assist the human body, to tissue grafting and then finally- to the use of a cell suspension to heal and regenerate a living tissue in the body has been the cynosure of the eyes of the research and medical fraternity. Each cautious step towards progress has been made with an abated breath. But finally, we can claim to have arrived into "*the age of Regenerative Medicine*."[1]

Throughout history, medicine has sought to facilitate or improve the intrinsic self-renewing ability of biological systems. Regenerative medicine is an emerging interdisciplinary field of research and clinical applications. It is expected to be a new way of treating injuries and diseases that uses ex vivo expanded cells including stem cells, engineered tissues and artificial organs. Thus, regenerative medicine is therefore focused on the development and application of innovative medical therapies to prevent further degeneration of organs and subsequently repair, replace, restore and regenerate the damaged or diseased organs, make tissue engineered constructs or catalyze self renewal of the organs or parts of it. It uses a combination of several technological approaches that move it beyond traditional transplantation and replacement therapies. These approaches may include, but are not limited to, the use of soluble molecules, gene therapy, stem cell transplantation, tissue engineering and the programming of cell and tissue types. [2]

Current treatments for various degenerative disorders rely on surgical interventions and drugs that modulate the system, but these have their own limitations when it comes to regeneration of damaged tissues and cells. To address this shortcoming, cell-based therapies are gaining importance. Among the different types of stem cells studied adult stem cells such as mesenchymal stem cells (MSCs) are most widely researched for their therapeutic applications. Adult stem cells have generated great amount of interest amongst the scientific community for their potential therapeutic applications for unmet medical needs. Haematopoietic stem cells and MSCs are the two widely studied and characterized adult stem cells.

Mesenchymal stem cells as a choice for cell-based therapies in Regenerative medicine are becoming very clear. There are increasing amount of literature indicating its usefulness in clinical applications which is very encouraging. Within the bone marrow stroma there exists a subset of non haematopoietic cells referred to as mesenchymal stem cell or mesenchymal progenitor cells. These cells can be ex vivo expanded and induced either in vitro or in vivo, to terminally differentiate into osteoblasts, chrondrocytes, adipocytes, tenocytes, myotubes, neural cells, and haematopoeitic supporting stroma. [3] The multipotential of these cells, their easy isolation and culture as well as their high ex vivo expansion potential make these cells an attractive tool capable of playing a role in a wide range of clinical applications in the context of both cell and gene therapy.[4]

MSCs have generated a great deal of interest because of their potential use in regenerative medicine and tissue engineering and there are some dramatic examples, derived from both pre-clinical and clinical studies that illustrate their therapeutic value. This chapter summarizes the usefulness regarding the potential clinical use of MSCs in various applications. As new methods are developed, there are several aspects to the implanted cell–host interaction that need to be addressed before we can fully understand the underlying mechanisms. These include the host immune response to implanted cells, the homing mechanisms that guide delivered cells to a site of injury and the differentiation in vivo of implanted cells under the influence of local signals. Both pre-clinical and clinical studies offer dramatic examples that illustrate the therapeutic value of MSCs. This chapter will describe the characteristics of MSCs derived from various sources, as well as some of the many clinical applications that are currently being evaluated. [5]

Different Sources for MSCs

Human MSCs were first identified in postnatal bone marrow and later in a variety of other human adult tissues, including muscle, connective tissue, skin, adipose tissue, perichondrium, trabecular bone, placenta, umbilical cord blood, and umbilical cord. [6] This explains why many researchers have chosen to work with MSCs from the traditional and nonconventional sources. Currently, BM represents the main source of MSCs (BMMSCs) for both experimental and clinical studies, but with limitations. Bone marrow - mesenchymal stem cells have been used in several clinical trials in various domains, such as, cardiology, neurology, and so on, with its limitations in the autologous settings, as it represents 0.01-0.001% of the nucleated cells in the adult human marrow. Allogeneic BMMSCs are also under research and in an advance phase of clinical trial for its application in cartilage injury and Crohn's disease. Besides, bone marrow aspiration being an invasive procedure, its frequency and differentiation capacity decline with age, reducing their therapeutic potential.

Hence, to overcome these limitations there is a need for an alternative source, which is easily available, noncontroversial, and could generate a higher number of MSCs. Therefore, the search for alternative sources of MSCs is of significant value. Of these different sources, human umbilical cord blood, cord tissue and adipose tissue could successfully replace BM as a source for MSCs.

In the study conducted by us, we have successfully isolated, expanded, and compared the MSCs from three sources such as Adipose tissue (AT), Cord blood (CB) and Cord matrix (CM) with the BM, which is a well-studied and accessible source of MSCs. [7] The MSCs from three different sources have been compared for their common cell surface epitopes and multilineage differentiation potentials to mesodermal and ectodermal lineages. [8] Our study has shown that CM can address the issue of availability, as it is an abundant and easily available source. MSCs can be easily derived from CMs, which have high expansion potential. As these MSCs do not express MHC class II antigens, they can, along with their immunomodulatory mechanisms, address several immunological issues in a clinical set up. In the recent past, MSCs have been used for CD34 expansion and GVHD prevention too. [9]

Identification and Characterization of MSCs

Plastic-adherent multipotent cells, capable of differentiating into bone, cartilage and fat cells (among others), can be isolated from many adult tissue types. However, even if isolated by density-gradient fractionation, they remain a heterogeneous mixture of cells with varying proliferation and differentiation potentials. Although acceptable for cell-based therapeutic applications, a rigorous understanding of the MSC requires a better definition of what an MSC is. Many attempts have been made to develop a cell-surface antigen profile for the better purification and identification of MSCs. Particularly important is whether MSCs isolated from different tissues are identifiable by the same immunophenotype. Most of the studies focused on MSCs from human bone marrow, but some examined MSCs from other organs. There is a surprisingly small amount of variation between populations, even among cells isolated from different sources.

Negative Markers

There is a consensus that MSCs do not express CD11b (an immune cell marker), glycophorin-A (an erythroid lineage marker), or CD45 (a marker of all hematopoietic cells). CD34, the primitive hematopoietic stem cell (HSC) marker, is rarely expressed in human MSCs, although it is positive in mice. CD31 (expressed on endothelial and hematopoietic cells) and CD117 (a hematopoietic stem/progenitor cell marker) are almost always absent from human and mouse MSCs. [10]

Positive Markers

Stro-1 is by far the best-known MSC marker. The cell population negative for Stro-1 is not capable of forming colonies (that is, it does not contain CFU-Fs). [11] Negative selection against glycophorin-A, together with selection of strongly Stro-1-positive cells, enriches CFU-Fs in harvested bone marrow cells to a frequency of 1 in 10. [12] Stro-1- positive cells can become HSC-supporting fibroblasts, smooth muscle cells, adipocytes, osteoblasts, and chondrocytes [13], which is consistent with the functional role of MSCs. In addition, expression of Stro-1 distinguishes between two cultured populations of MSCs that have different homing and HSC-supportive capacities [14]. CD106, or VCAM-1 (vascular cell adhesion molecule-1), is expressed on blood vessel endothelial and adjacent cells, consistent with a perivascular location of MSCs. It is likely to be functional in MSCs because it is involved in cell adhesion, chemotaxis, and signal transduction, and has been implicated in rheumatoid arthritis [15]. CD106 singles out 1.4% of Stro-1-positive cells, increasing the CFU-F frequency to 1 in 3, which are all high Stro-1-expressing cells and are the only Stro-1-positive cells that form colonies and show stem cell characteristics such as multipotentiality, expression of telomerase, and high proliferation *in vitro* Taken together, these data suggest that Stro-1 and CD106 combine to make a good human MSC marker.

MSCs, as defined by the International Society for Cellular Therapy (ISCT), are multipotent, spindle like plastic adherent cells capable of self-renewal and possess the ability to differentiate *in vitro* to bone, cartilage and adipose tissues. Phenotypic characterization studies of MSCs have shown that these cells express CD73, CD105, CD90, CD29 and CD44 cell surface antigens, and are negative for CD34, CD45, CD31, CD14, human leukocyte

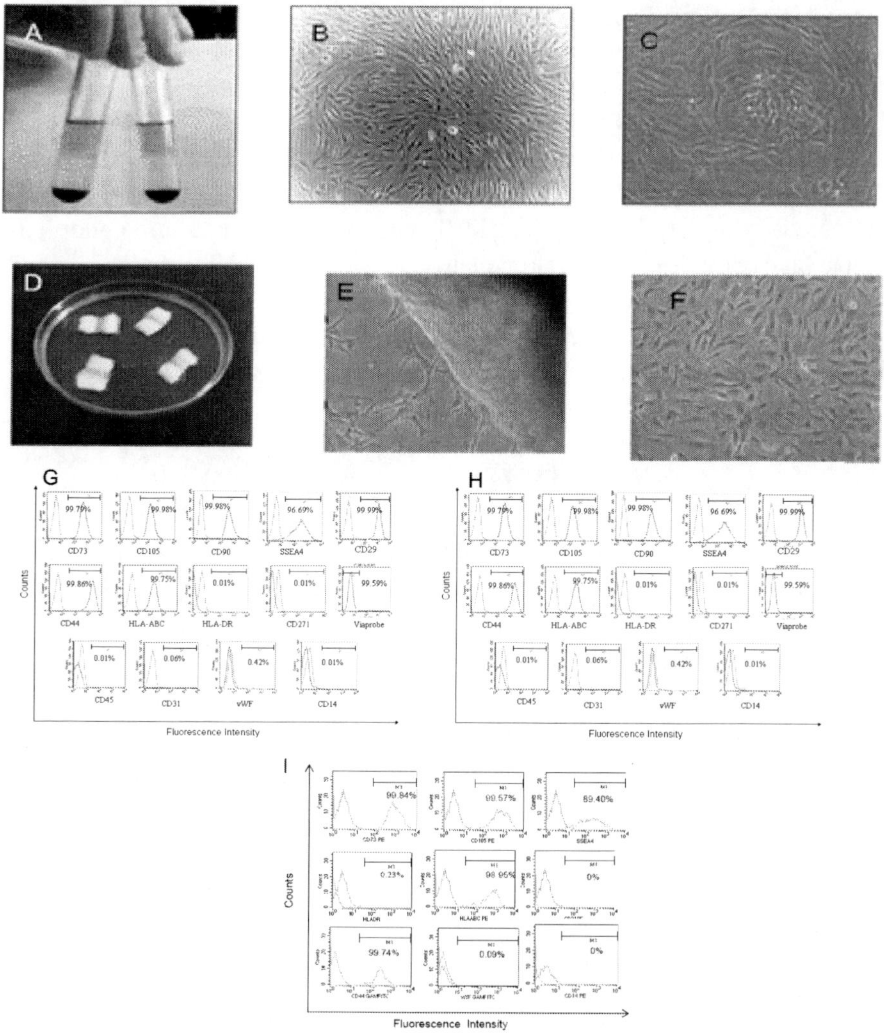

Figure 1. A: Processing of thc Bone marrow and cord blood samples for Mononuclear cell separation to obtain the MSCs. The Mononuclear fraction is obtained by density gradient separation. B: Morphology of the human bone marrow derived mesenchymal stem cells. C: Morphology of the human cord blood derived mesenchymal stem cells D: Explant culture method for derivation of mesenchymal stem cells from human umbilical cord tissue. E: MSCs growing from the cord explants. F: Confluent layer of MSCs derived from human umbilical cord. G, H, I: Characterization of the human umbilical cord derived MSCs, human bone marrow derived MSCs and human umbilical cord blood derived MSCs respectively. These MSCs were 98 - 99% positive for all the MSC markers and cell adhesion molecules and were negative for hematopoietic markers.

antigen (HLA)-class II antigens and von Willebrand factor. Recently some interesting molecules were described which may be useful to identify MSC (sub) populations (CD271, GD2, CD49a, W7C5, W8B2, C15, CDCP1, CD340, CD349, SSEA1/4). However, a distinct exclusively MSC-restricted marker has yet to be identified. Furthermore, the cellular shape by itself is not sufficient to determine the cells because the morphology of MSC may vary from spindle shape to broad trapezoid shape depending on culture conditions and passages. Due to the heterogeneity of MSC-like cell populations and biased sample preparations, it is necessary to standardize the characterization of MSC. For this purpose, a useful approach is application of the minimal criteria for defining MSC which have been published by the ISCT [16].

MSC Differentiation

The identification of specific signaling networks and 'master' regulatory genes that govern unique MSC differentiation lineages remains a challenge. The ability to modulate biological effectors to maintain a desired differentiation program, or possibly to prevent spurious differentiation of MSCs, is needed for effective clinical application, as in tissue engineering and regeneration. Some of the recently discovered lineage-restrictive molecular regulators and their mechanisms of action are reviewed here. *In vitro* differentiation studies have shown that MSCs could differentiate to additional cell types encompassing mesodermal (myocytes and tendon), as well as cells of ectodermal (neurons) and endodermal (hepatocytes, pancreatic) lineages. Treatment with growth factors such as epithelial growth factor and brain-derived neurotrophic factor or chemical products such as dimethyl sulfoxide and butylated hydroxyanisole induced the bone marrow stroma cells to exhibit a neuronal phenotype. In addition to osteoblastic, adipocytic and chondrocytic differentiation, MSC acquired an unexpected phenotype after their exposure to different factors *in vitro*. Various studies induced MSC differentiation into neurons and glial cells. After *in vitro* neural differentiation cells demonstrated an assortment of neuronal and glial markers, such as neuronspecific enolase (NSE), neuronal nuclear antigen (NeuN), neurofilament M (NF-M), tau, glial fibrillary acidic protein (GFAP) and adopted neuronal and glial morphology. Researchers found that BMMSCs expressed germline, ectodermal, endodermal, in addition to mesodermal, genes prior to the induced neural differentiation and hypothesized that neural differentiation involves modulated expression of these genes.

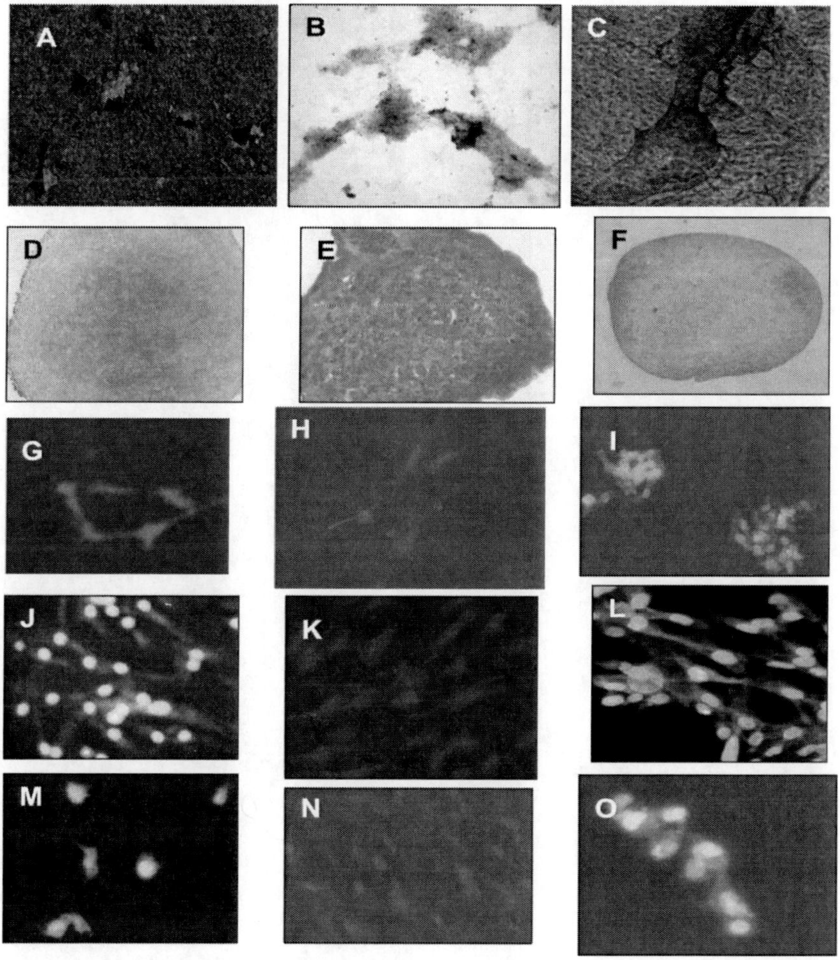

Figure 2. Differentiation of mesenchymal stem cells to osteocytes as detected byVon kossa staining of (A) BMMSC; (B) CBMSC; (C) CMMSC Differentiation of mesenchymal stem cells to chondrocytes as detected by Safranin O staining Immunohistochemical staining of pellet cultures from different sources for detection of proteoglycans of (D) BMMSC; (E) CBMSC; (F) UCMSC. Neuronal differentiation of expanded confirmed by Immunofluorescence for detection of Nestin (G) BMMSC; (H) CBMSC; (I) UCMSC.Neuronal differentiation of expanded confirmed by Immunofluorescence for detection of Beta tubulin (J) BMMSC; (K) CBMSC; (L) UCMSC. Neuronal differentiation of expanded confirmed by Immunofluorescence for detection of NeuN (M) BMMSC; (N) CBMSC; (O) UCMSC.

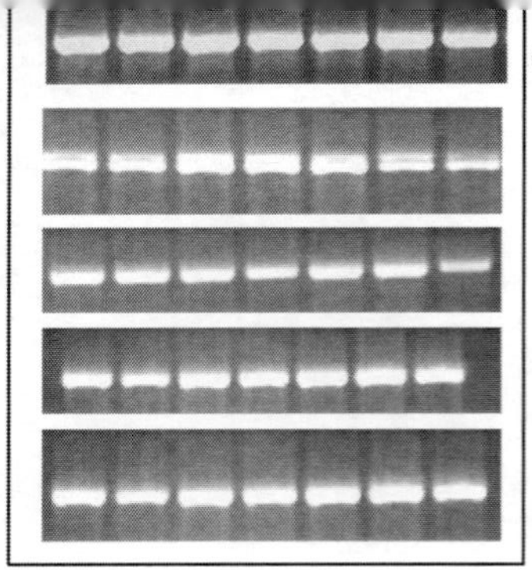

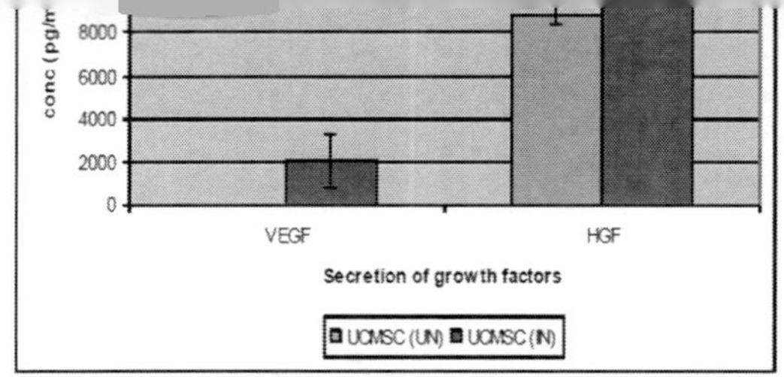

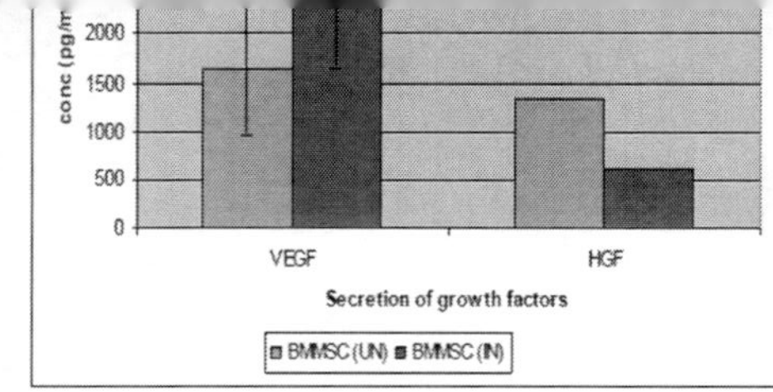

Cell Type	VEGF (pg/ml)	HGF (pg/ml)
UCMSCs (UN)	0.67	8838
UCMSCs (IN)	2061	12771
BMMSCs (UN)	1647	1342
BMMSCs (IN)	2291	624
HFF	ND	ND

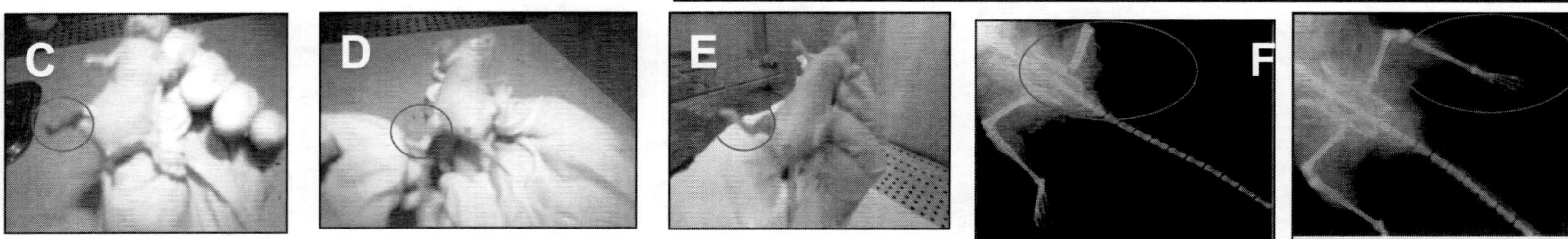

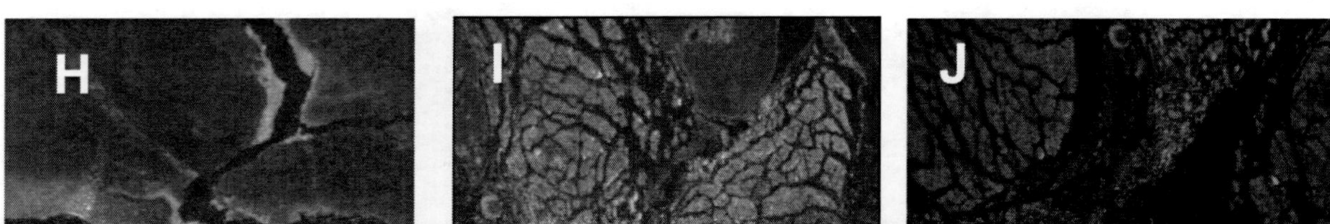

and HFF (Lane 7) were analyzed for genes such as VEGF,HGF, TGF□1 and bFGF. UCMSCs showed a good expression of all the genes which were analyzed. BMMSCs and dermal fibroblasts also were found to be positive for all theabove genes. B) Analysis of VEGF and HGF secretion by the MSCs post induction with TNFα: UCMSCs and BMMSCs were induced with TNFα and secretion of VEGF and HGF were checked by ELISA. The growth factors secreted by the uninduced (UN) and induced (IN) MSCs were compared. The UN UCMSCs did not show any secretion of VEGF but upon induction a significant amount of VEGF was secreted which was almost equivalent to the BMMSCs. HGF secretion in the UCMSCs was also elevated post induction. The IN BMMSCs did not show any significant difference in the secretion of both these factors as compared to the UN cells. Transplantation of the mesenchymal stem cells into the hind limbs of the ischemic limb disease (ILD) mice model and contrast imaging of the transplanted limb. C. HFF injected ILD mice showing necrosis of the ligated limb. The degenerated limb was then shed off within a week of transplantation of the HFF cells. D) Umbilical cord derived mesenchymal stem cells (UCMSCs) were injected into the ligated limb of the ILD mice showed improvement of the limb within 48 hrs. The necrosis seen due to the ligation of the femoral artery was improved by the UCMSC injection. E) Bone marrow derived MSCs (BMMSCs) treated ILD mice also showed improvement of the ligated limb post transplantation of the cells within a week. Skiagram of the hind Limbs of the Nude Mice after the injection of Iodine Contrast Agent (Urographin™) viewed in Kodak In-Vivo Image Analyzer (35kVp). ILD Model- Control (F) Control animal is showing degeneration of the femoral artery. The leg from the stifle joint has sloughed off due to stoppage of blood circulation (G) UCMSC injected into the ILD animal model is showing regeneration of the collateral blood circulation12 weeks after MSC injection in which the femoral artery was permanently ligated. Histological analysis of the muscle section of the ischemic limb disease (ILD) mice. H) DiI labeled HFF injected into the limb of ILD mice. The mice injected with the cells lost the limb in a week. The muscles show total disintegration of the muscle bundles. I &J) DiI labeled umbilical cord derived mesenchymal stem cells (UCMSCs) injected into the ILD mice restored the limb of the ILD mice which was ligated. Muscle section of the UCMSCs and BMMSCs injected limb shows good muscle integration which was similar to the normal muscle.

In addition, MAPC were found to differentiate into endothelial cells. The liver too, may perhaps be regenerated by differentiated MSC. Rat MSC were stimulated to differentiate into cells with hepatocyte-like phenotypes after treatment with HGF. MSCs have been reported to differentiate into various epithelial cell types after systemic administration in vivo. MSCs have been shown to differentiate into retinal pigment epithelial cells [17,18], skin epithelial cells [19], sebaceous duct cells [20] and tubular epithelial cells in kidney . [21, 22] The epithelial differentiation of MSCs was assessed based on their distribution within the tubuli, alignment within the epithelial areas showing well-defined brush borders and expression of epithelial specific cells. [23].

Preclinical Studies

Angiogenesis

We have demonstrated that MSCs secrete several important arteriogenic cytokines where they orchestrate processes that ultimately lead to collateral vessel growth. This is a comparative study between MSC derived from umbilical cord and bone marrow for their role in the treatment of peripheral vascular diseases. A higher expression of mesenchymal as well as pluripotent stem cell marker such as SSEA4 was seen in the UCMSCs demonstrating its naivety and primitiveness in comparison to the BMMSCs. In addition, these cells also expressed mRNAs that encode for the genes related to endothelial cell lineages. *In vitro* functional studies also showed UCMSCs secreting elevated levels of angiogeneic factors such as vascular endothelial growth factor (VEGF) and hepatocyte growth factor (HGF). VEGF is a positive regulator and plays a crucial role in angiogenesis. HGF secreted by the mesenchymal cells acts as a multifunctional cytokine and plays a central role in angiogenesis and tissue regeneration. A marked difference was observed in the cytokine expression pattern between the two types of MSCs. In the uninduced state, the UCMSCs did not express any VEGF but showed higher levels of HGF while BMMSCs secreted both VEGF and HGF in the uninduced state. UCMSCs upon stimulation with TNFα, the expression of VEGF increased significantly along with the HGF levels whereas reduced level of the cytokines was observed in the BMMSCs post stimulation.

Many cytokines are elevated during conditions of ischemia or endotoxemia and stimulating stem cells with TNF or LPS creates a harsh condition in the *in vitro* conditions. This suggests that the UCMSCs being from a neonatal source plays a significant role in mobilizing cytokines and stimulating angiogenesis during ischemia. Efficacy studies with both the types of MSCs were performed by injecting equal numbers into the abductor muscles of the ischemic hind limb. MSCs significantly enhanced perfusion of ischemic tissue and collateral remodeling, lessened tissue damage and improved limb function [24]. Animal studies have provided a useful tool for defining a number of diverse potential applications for MSCs. It has been demonstrated that cultured mesenchymal cells could home to the bone marrow in non-human primates. The ability of culture-expanded human mesenchymal cells to contribute to the functional repair of a skeletal defect has also been examined using a variety of animal models. MSCs repaired an 8 mm defect in a rat femur when placed into a porous cylinder which was then implanted into the bone. After 8 weeks, the defect containing the MSC-loaded implant completely healed, while the defects containing cylinders filled with control cell populations failed to heal successfully. These studies indicate that culture-expanded MSCs are able to both persist and contribute to de novo bone formation *in vivo*. Studies in sheep have addressed the possibility of using mesenchymal cells to enhance engraftment of transplanted hematopoietic cells. In utero co-transplantation of fetal sheep with human bone marrow stromal cells along with human HSC enhanced long-term engraftment of human HSCs [25]. Transplantation of unprocessed whole bone marrow cells has been shown to restore microenvironmental function, suggesting that unprocessed bone marrow contains stromal precursors as well as hematopoietic precursors that contribute to hematopoietic regeneration following transplantation. Given the recent finding that osteoblasts are a crucial component of the HSC niche, it is likely that transplanted MSCs serve to reconstitute the hematopoietic microenvironment.

Recent studies have shown that BMMSCs improve neurological deficits when transplanted into animal models of neurological disorders. The transdifferentiation potential of MSCs into neurons *in vitro* has been reported by many researchers. Cytokines, growth factors, neurotrophins, and retinoic acid have been used to promote neural cell induction and differentiation both *in vivo* and *in vitro*. Several clinical applications of MSCs would theoretically involve the administration of MSCs by the intravenous route.

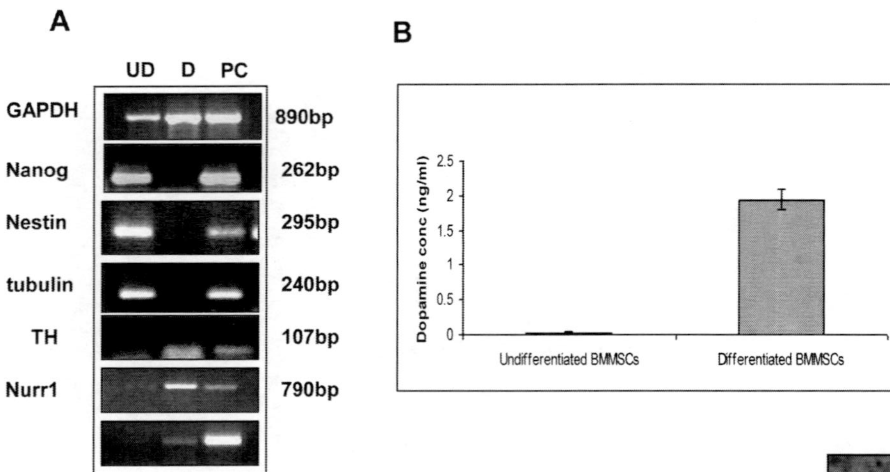

C

	Mean Dopamine secretion (ng/ml)	SD
Undifferentiate d BMMSCs	0.03	0.01
Differentiated BMMSCs	1.95	0.14
p value	0.000102845	

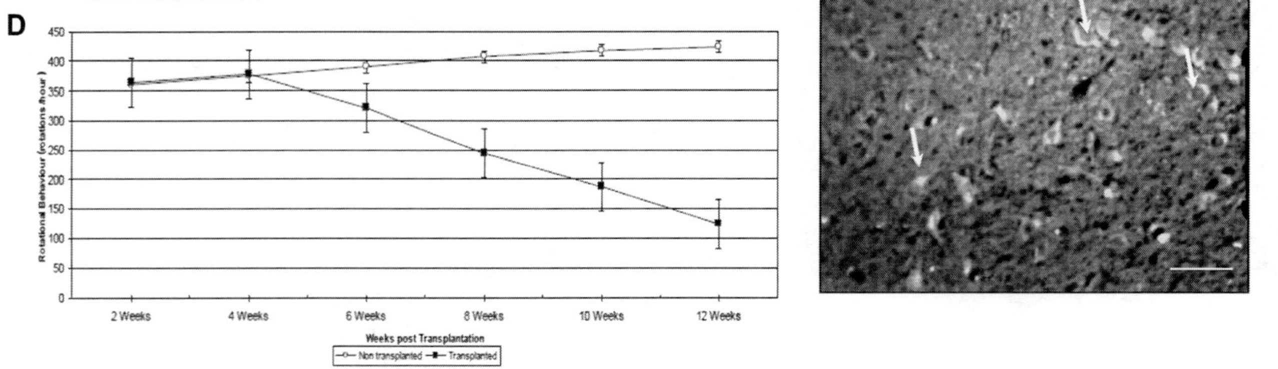

Figure 4. A) Gene expression studies of neuron specific markers by Reverse Transcriptase PCR (RT-PCR). Undifferentiated (UD) and differentiated cells (D) were checked for neuron specific genes, with Ntera 2 cells as positive control. Undifferentiated cells expressed stem cell marker Nanog and neuron specific genes Nestin and b tubulin. The differentiated cells expressed neuronal and dopaminergic specific genes

specific genes such as NFM and Nurr1, TH. B) & C) Measurement of dopamine released into the culture supernatant. Samples were separated on reverse phase nucleosil C18 column and detected with an electrochemical detector. Dopamine levels were calculated using external dopamine standards injected immediately before and after each experiment. Concentrationof dopamine released by differentiated BMMSCs was significantly higher (1.95 ng/ml) compared to the undifferentiated BMMSCs (0.03 ng/ml), as tabulated in the figure. D) Behavioural analysis of the PD animals injected with BMMSCs expanded in xenofree medium. The number of apomorphine-induced rotations per h wascounted in the transplanted and non-transplanted animals. The graph compares the rotations in the transplanted and non-transplanted animals at 2, 4, 6, 8, 10 and12weeks. Transplanted animals showed reduction in rotations from 4 weeks post-transplantation. The transplanted animals showed continuous and significant improvement as the weeks progressed. E) Immunohistochemistry of brain sections of PD induced rats. Transverse section of the PD rat brain 12 weeks post transplantation shows positive staining for both TH (FITC) and human nuclei (Alexa 568) confirming the human origin of the transplanted cells as indicated by the arrows. Scale bars 50 mm.

However, limited data are available regarding the ultimate fate of systemically infused MSCs. Studies in rodents suggest a broad initial biodistribution followed by a limited capacity for sustained engraftment. In fetal sheep, MSCs undergo a wide tissue distribution and can differentiate into multiple mesenchymal tissues following peritoneal implantation. [26]

Solid Organ/Graft Transplantation

In immunocompetent baboons infusions of allogeneic MSCs prior to graft placement slightly prolonged survival of a skin allograft [27] and the same was demonstrated with a heart allograft in rats [28]. On the other hand, another study showed that MSCs did not affect survival of a vascularized heart transplant in rodents [29] and a study in a mouse model demonstrated that MSCs only improved heart transplant survival in the absence of HSCs, which might explain failures in other studies [30]. Still, in combination with immunosuppressive drugs, administration of MSCs has demonstrated some promising results. A short course of low---dose mycophenolate mofetil (MMP) [31] or rapamycin [32] combined with administration of MSCs prior to transplantation resulted in long---term graft survival in rat heart transplant models.

Kidney Failure

Several animal studies have demonstrated that injections of MSCs have beneficial effects in both acute and chronic kidney failure. Injected MSCs migrated towards the kidney and significantly improved renal function and regeneration, restored capillary defects, whereas they decreased apoptosis, renal injury scores and mortality [33, 34]. Observed effects were attributed to a reduction in the expression of pro-inflammatory cytokines (Il-1, TNFα INFγ, and NO synthase) and an increase in anti--- inflammatory cytokines (Il-10, bFGF, TGF? and Bcl-2) [32]. In contrast, infusion of MSCs did not affect renal injury in a sheep model, suggesting a species-dependent effect [35]. To the best of our knowledge, no clinical trials using MSCs to treat acute or chronic kidney failure have been completed so far, but one trial is currently ongoing and several others are scheduled.

Mycardial Infarction

Preliminary studies suggest that culture expanded MSC may possess that capacity to repair ischemic myocardial damage when directly injected into the infarct or the peri-infarct zone or intriguingly, when given by systemic infusion soon after induction of myocardial ischemia.

Although further refinement in these models is required, such results suggest a potential clinical application for MSC following myocardial infarction.

Preclinical models also suggest that the co-transplantation of stromal cells simultaneously with haematopoietic cells may enhance the engraftment potential of the haematopoietic cells .

In addition, MSC express a number of cytokines that are crucial for the support of haematopoiesis. [26]

Immunomodulatory and Trophic Effects of Therapeutic MSCs

Two distinctly different biological properties have made MSCs an attractive cell type for regeneration of damaged tissues. First, the MSCs have the ability to repopulate the damaged host tissue for repair and restoration and second, these cells exert their immunomodulatory and immunosuppressive properties to survive in allogeneic hosts.

In vivo observations after administration of MSC, like improvement of the outcome after allogeneic transplantations by promotion of hematopoietic engraftment and amelioration of graft versus- host disease as well as the amelioration of inflammatory response and improved clinical course in experimental allergic encephalomyelitis are impressive proofs for the immunomodulatory properties of MSC.

Regardless of the source from which these cells are isolated, MSCs have been shown to be immunologically naive and possess potent immunosuppressive properties, both *in vitro* and *in vivo* (36).

The multifaceted immunosuppressive activity of MSCs is mediated through cell surface-associated molecules as well as by soluble factors (37, 38).

MSCs do not induce allogeneic T-lymphocyte proliferation *in vitro* and also inhibit T-cell responses to mitogenic and antigenic stimuli. MSCs obtained from different sources can prevent the generation of antigen presenting cells that are critical for T-cell activation. CD4+CD25highFoxp3+ Treg cells have been implicated to have an important role in the regulation of immune response and inducing tolerance. Co-culture of MSCs with T cells, particularly in the presence of IFN-γ, has been shown to increase the generation of Treg cells.

Taken together, these results indicate that MSCs may have an important role in the regulation of Treg cell generation and tolerance induction. MSCs secrete immunomodulatory factors as well as reparative and regenerative factors.

Several studies have demonstrated differentiation of MSCs into different target cells, whereas low engraftment percentages, the short window in which MSCs exert their effects and the fact that conditioned medium alone often exerts similar responses underlines the particular importance of immunomodulatory and trophic mediators [39].

In 1996, it was noticed that isolated MSCs are able to secrete a broad spectrum of cytokines and growth factors that affect neighboring cells [40]. Specific growth factor panels and concentrations were found to vary between differently committed cells, but not between donors, donor age and donor health.

This trophic effect does not require differentiation of MSCs at target sites [41]. Work by Chen et al. showed that non activated human derived mesenchymal progenitor cells differ in their secretion proteome from more mature stromal cells, such as fibroblasts [42].

A higher expression was found in MSCs for most investigated growth factors, such as VEGF-A, ANG-1, TPO, hepatocyte growth factor (HGF), leukemia inhibitory factor (LIF), IGF, IGF-binding proteins-1, 2, 3,4, FGF 4, 6, 7, 9, and a number of other molecules such as leptin, fractalkine, neutrophil activating peptide-2 (NAP-2), macrophage inflammatory protein (MIP-1), and macrophage inflammatory protein, whilst a small number of cytokines (IL 6, 7, 8, 10) and growth factors (G-CSF, M-CSF, GM-CSF, SDF-1, SCF) was expressed at similar levels in both cell types. MSCs produce factors that decrease proliferation of CD4+ and CD8+ T cells, B cells, dendritic cells (DCs) and natural killer (NK) cells upon close contact [43,44]. MSCs can also polarize the differentiation and function of myeloid cells such as DCs [40]. MSC derived factors may therefore alter the maturation of antigen presenting cells [45], as well as the cytokine profile of various other cells.

Table 1. MSCs are positive for SDF-1, Flt-3, IL-6,ENA-78, GRO, Thrombopoetin, G-CSF, GM-CSF, SCF and LIF. Some of these factors are known to support growth and expansion of HSCs. The intensity of certain cytokines released by UCMSCs is clearly higher than those released by BMMSCs. UCMSCs released ENA-78, G-CSF, MCP-2, EGF, thrombopoietin and LIF but BMMSCs did not secrete these cytokines and growth factors as shown in the table. The expression of GM-CSF, SDF-1, Angiogenin, Flt-3 ligand and HGF secreted by BMMSCs was comparatively lower to that produced by UCMSCs. These results, though qualitative in nature, may suggest that UCMSCs obtained from the fetal cord tissue, release important cytokines and chemokines essential to support growth and expansion of other cell types

Cytokine	UCMSCs	BMMSCs
Positive control	+++	+++
Negative control	-	-
ENA-78	+	-
G-CSF	+	-
GM-CSF	++	+
GRO	++	++
IL-6	+++	+++
MCP-1	++	++
MCP-2	+	-
MCP-3	+++	+
M-CSF	+	+
SCF	+	+
SDF-1	++	+
EGF	+	-
IGF-1	+	-
Angiogenin	+++	+
Thrombopoietin	++	-
FGF-4	+	+
FGF-6	+	-
FGF-7	+	-
FGF-9	+	-
Flt-3 ligand	++	+
HGF (hepatocyte growth factor)	+++	+
LIF	++	-

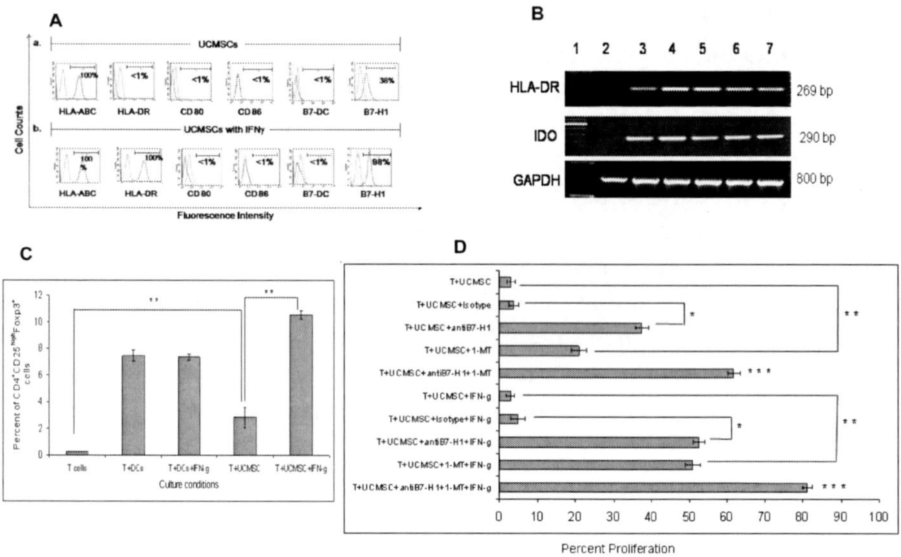

Figure 5. A) Immunological phenotype of UCMSCs a. Expression of co-stimulatory molecules on UCMSCs. UCMSCs were stained with directly conjugated antibodies against HLA-ABC, HLA-DR, CD80, CD86, B7-DC and B7-H1 and were analyzed by flow cytometry.b. UCMSCs were stained after 5 days of treatment with IFN-γ (10ng/ml) with the same antibodies. B) Semi quantitative reverse transcriptase polymerase chain reaction (RT-PCR) for detection of IDO and HLA-DR mRNA in UCMSC samples. Kinetics of HLA-DR and IDO gene expression of one representative UCMSC sample following IFN-γ treatment for 5 days. Similar to IDO, expression of HLA-DR mRNA was observed only after IFN-γ treatment. GAPDH mRNA was used as a positive control. Lane 1 : 100bp Marker, Lane 2: UCMSC day 0, Lane 3: UCMSC + IFN-γ, day 1, Lane 4: UCMSC + IFN-γ, day 2, Lane 5: UCMSC + IFN-γ, day 3, Lane 6: UCMSC + IFN-γ, day 4, Lane 7: UCMSC + IFN-γ, day 5. C) Induction of regulatory T cells by UCMSCs. Peripheral blood T cells obtained from normal donors were cultured for 5 days alone, with mDCs, with mDCs + IFN-γ (10ng/ml), with UCMSCs and with UCMSCs + IFN-γ. The T cells were harvested, labeled with antibodies to CD4, CD25 and Foxp3 and analyzed by flow cytometry. D) Ablation of UCMSC induced T cell suppression by anti B7-H1 antibody and 1-MT. Percent inhibition of T cell suppression is shown for various conditions used and is expressed as mean ± SD.

They may change the pro-inflammatory profile of T-helper1 (TH1) cells towards a TH2 cells anti inflammatory profile and decrease the secretion of inflammatory proteins, such as tumor necrosis factor-a (TNFα) and interferon g (INFγ) by DCs and T cells, respectively [47]. The factors identified to mediate these processes include short lived metabolites produced by enzymes such as: prostaglandin E2 (PGE2), a product of cyclic oxide synthase (COX) [47]; kynurenine, a product of indoleamine 2,3 dioxygenase

(IDO) [48]; biliverdin and carbon monoxide, the products of hemoxigenase-1 (HO-1); and nitric oxide, the product of nitric oxide synthase (NOS) [49]; but also cytokines such as IL-10 and TGFβ [46], and a number of other factors such as HGF [45], LIF [50], and soluble human leukocyte---antigen-G5 (sHLA-G5) [51, 52] were identified as possible immunomodulatory mediators. More recently described molecules with immunoregulatory functions include CCL2 (MCP-1), galectin-1 (GAL-1) and TNF α, stimulated gene/protein 6 (TSG-6) [53].

Clinical Applications

MSCs are currently studied as treatment for inflammatory diseases such as graft-versus host disease, but also as treatment for myocardial infarct and solid organ transplantation. In addition, MSCs are investigated for their use in tissue engineering applications, in which their differentiation plays an important role. Given the promising features of the adult stem cells for the development of new cell therapies, researchers in the field of mesenchymal progenitors have pursued a broad range of investigations to give impulse to their therapeutic utilization. However, a main issue to be resolved is whether mesenchymal progenitors are transplantable, and in addition what type of progenitor (uncommitted versus committed) is transplantable. These questions will help to decide whether direct loading (injection or implant) or systemic infusion is the best route of mesenchymal progenitor delivery. The former case is probably best suited with clinical strategy oriented to augment local repair or regeneration of bone [54, 55, 56], cartilage [57], or tendon [58]. On the other side, blood delivery of mesenchymal progenitors may be useful in recovering not only a local, but also systemic dysfunction of a tissue by re-starting their own developmental program. Particularly, in the case of bone marrow one may speculate that the infusion of mesenchymal progenitors followed by selective homing into the marrow stromal sites can result in the increase or improvement of the function of haematopoietic-supporting stroma, which in turn may facilitate engraftment and differentiation of haematopoietic stem cells. [59,60]

The issue of transplantability has been addressed in several studies; however, results are rather contradictory in establishing the origin (host or donor) of mesenchymal progenitors after allogeneic transplantation of marrow harvests. Contradiction probably arises from the use of different experimental conditions, among them procedures to harvest the marrow, methods to type and measure progenitor content in marrow harvest and patient's marrow status to which cells are transplanted. In addition, it appears essential to take into account whether the material to be transplanted has to be ex vivo expanded to increase the number of progenitors. This may be an important issue, since progenitor stemness and function diverge as cells are subcultivated. In the haematopoietic and muscle systems it has been demonstrated that stemness of the grafted cells determines the long or short term repopulation of the damaged tissue. [61, 62] It has yet to be established whether the same occurs after transplantation of ex vivo expanded mesenchymal progenitors.

The first clinical trials reported have revealed that the systemic infusion of ex vivo expanded mesenchymal progentiors is feasible and safe in the short term.[59, 63] On the other hand it has been demonstrated that allogeneic bone marrow transplantation (considered as common source of haematopoietic and mesenchymal progenitors) in children with osteogenesis imperfecta results in impressive histological changes in trabecular bone., which are indicative of new dense bone formation. In addition increased growth rate and reduced frequencies of bone fracture were also observed. These changes detected 3 months after marrow transplantation, were associated with the engraftment of functional mesenchymal progenitors from the transplanted marrow. [64, 65]

In 2005, a clinical trial was performed, in which 35 patients with complex perianal fistulas received either fibrin glue or fibrin glue with adipose derived MSCs. In the control group only 16% of the patients showed fistula healing, whereas in the group receiving MSCs, 71% showed healing. [66]

Myocardial Infarction

In 2001, Orlic et al showed that transplantation of Lin-kit+ bone marrow cells resulted in the formation of new myocardium, consisting of infused cells. [67] Later, adipose tissue--derived progenitor cells were shown to engraft into the myocardium and to express both cardiac and endothelial markers. A study by Zisa et al. showed beneficial effects of conditioned medium on heart function after myocardial infarcts (MI), which was attributed to either VEGF, IGF and monocyte chemotactic protein 1 (MCP1). [68] Other known cardio protective growth factors include FGFs, HGF and VEGF, which are produced by skeletal muscle cells, and whose over expression was shown to benefit the myocardium. [69] Injection of MSCs resulted in elevated levels of circulating HGF, LIF and granulocyte/macrophage colony-stimulating factor (GM-CSF), as well as the HGF, IGF2 and VEGF levels in the myocardium. MSCs appear to exert beneficial effects by attracting progenitor cells and by triggering growth factor secretion by host cells. [70] Regardless the underlying mechanisms, intracoronary administration of bone marrow derived cells for MI has been tested in several clinical trials, with various outcomes.

Meta analysis of 13 clinical trials, with a total of 811 patients, concluded that stem cell therapy improves left ventricular ejection fraction (LVEF), reduces LV end systolic volume and myocardial lesion area. [71] Preliminary clinical study including 10 patients, demonstrated that MSCs can be safely applied in chronic as well as acute wounds and that wound healing correlated with the amount of infused MSCs. [72]

Neuroprotective Effects of MSCs

In a small pilot study with five stroke patients some improvements after injection of MSCs were demonstrated, but due to the small study number, no definitive conclusions could be made [73]. Similarly, a small, uncontrolled study with seven patients for treatment of Parkinson's disease showed encouraging results, but due to the lack of a control group and the small study number no conclusions could be drawn [74]. Another pilot study for the treatment of ALS including seven patients, showed a trend towards slowing down of muscular strength decline, but again no conclusions could be drawn. A somewhat larger study with 21 patients for the treatment of MS and ALS, reported fever as a small side effect of MSC injection, but no major adverse effects. They also showed slight increase in functional behavior [75]. Due to these encouraging results, several clinical trials are currently on the way or scheduled to test the use of MSCs in Parkinson's disease, spinal cord injury, stroke, ALS and Multiple Sclerosis.

Graft versus Host Disease

In 2008, 55 patients were infused with 1-5 doses of expanded bone marrow derived MSCs in a phase II clinical trial. 30 patients showed a complete response, 9 patients a partial response and 16 patients showed stable or progressive disease. Patients with complete response showed higher survival than patients with partial or no response [76]. It was also reported on a single patient case of a 9-year old boy with treatment---resistant grade IV gastrointestinal GvHD, where intravenous infusions of *ex vivo* expanded MSCs resulted in complete recovery of the gut and liver [77]. In another clinical trial performed by Osiris Therapeutics Inc., 3-21 intravenous infusions of culture expanded allogeneic hMSCs resulted in complete remission in 7 out of 12 children after 1 month, and after 6 months, 95% of these children were still alive. [78]

Conclusion

The versatile and tunable differentiation potential of MSCs in conjunction with their ability to secrete various trophic factors and modulate the recipient's immune system makes them a promising cell source in regenerative medicine. Most of the research has been done in the last decade focusing on characterizing MSCs derived from various sources and understanding their differentiation potential. However, the complex mechanisms and pathways with which MSCs support repair are far from fully understood. While the therapeutic testing of these cells has progressed well, there are still many questions to be addressed concerning the role of endogenous populations of stem cells in the adult, and the functions of various stem cell niches. In addition, there are several aspects to the implanted cell–host interaction that need to be addressed as we attempt to understand the mechanisms underlying these therapies. Firstly, host responses to allogeneic MSC therapy need to be defined. Secondly, little is known about the mechanisms that direct homing and engraftment of implanted cells and thirdly, the response of MSCs to local differentiation signals in vivo has not been clarified.

Human clinical data show a wide range of potential applications for MSCs. There is overwhelming evidence of their usefulness in regenerative medicine, tissue engineering, and immune therapy. Although adult MSC transformation can be observed *in vitro* and in animals, no malignant transformation of implanted cells has been reported in patients. Infusion of allogeneic MSCs appears to be free of major hazardous events and does not raise any ethical issues, such as those related to use of human embryonic stem cells. MSCs migrate to sites of tissue injury in response to local signals, with critical phenotypic changes and intense paracrine activity that contributes to the reparative process. Among the MSCs, allogeneic MSCs have unique immunomodulatory properties. Their immunosuppressive capabilities without evidence of immunosuppressive toxicity at a global level define their application in the treatment of diseases in which the pathogenesis involves uncontrolled activity of the immune system.

MSCs possess important immunoregulatory and immunosuppressive properties. The inhibition of T-cell stimulation by MSCs is simultaneously governed by a cell surface-associated negative regulator, B7-H1, as well as by the tryptophan-catabolizing enzyme, IDO, even under inflammatory conditions. In addition, suppression of monocyte to DC differentiation, maturation as well as induction of Treg cell generation suggests the wide array of immunomodulatory function of these cells. [79] These immunological properties of MSCs need to be critically evaluated in *in vivo* disease models. Nevertheless, possession of such unique immunoregulatory functions by MSCs may be extremely relevant in the intervention of T cell-mediated autoimmune diseases and for prevention of rejection after transplantation cases in which the pathogenesis involves uncontrolled activity of the immune system. [80]

MSCs thus represent a promising tool for potential therapeutic applications characterized by cell loss or cell degeneration. Making MSCs available for regenerative medicine applications in adequate quantities and at the right time is a challenge. Clinical situations will demand MSCs with dependable quality and quantity to treat various disorders represented by cellular degeneration. [81] As we will soon move from autologous therapies to allogeneic therapies, the challenge will be the availability of a non-controversial supply of starting material, in adequate numbers, to address the ever-increasing number of patients the world over, who will look forward to this mode of therapy. A major stumbling block in the translation of this technology into the clinic is the use of animal sera or serum components in the culture media used for culturing MSC. Currently MSC are being cultured in FBS-containing media and being of animal origin, this is unsuitable for infusion into human beings. To overcome this limitation, attempts have been made to culture bone marrow stromal cells by substituting FBS with human AB serum .With cord blood serum (CBS) this will not be a problem since sera from multiple donors can be pooled to generate enough quantities of serum for large scale cultures. Our study shows that human cord blood serum can be used across species and the growth-promoting activity of human cord blood serum is not restricted to human MSC, although the efficiency of growth promotion may vary between species. Thus the use of CBS solves the issue of infusion of xenogeneic sera into humans with a unique solution that will be of utmost importance in the field of regenerative medicine [81, 82].

MSCs could turn out to be an ideal source for cell replacement therapy for several good biological properties they possess. Their self-renewing ability, multilineage developmental potential, easy availability and unique properties of plasticity are some of the properties that may be useful in combating various degenerative diseases. Thus, MSCs could be a likely alternative to fetal neuronal tissue or embryonic cells in replacing the damaged tissues for several degenerative diseases.

References

[1] Greenwood HL, Thorsteinsdottir H, Perry G et al., (2006). Regenerative medicine: new opportunities for developing countries. *Int. J. Biotechnol.*, 8(1-2), 60-77.

[2] Alhadlaq A and Mao JJ. (2004). Mesenchymal stem cells: Isolation and therapeutics. *Stem Cells and Development*, 13, 436-448.

[3] Bruder SP, Fink DJ and Caplan AI. (1994). Mesenchymal stem cells in bone development, bone repair, and skeletal regeneration therapy. *Journal of Cellular Biochemistry*, 56, 283-294.

[4] Heike T and Nakahata T. (2004). Stem cell plasticity in the hematopoietic system. *International Journal of Hematology*, 79, 7-14.

[5] Barry FP and Murphy MM. (2004). Mesenchymal stem cells: clinical applications and biological characterization. *The International Journal of Biochemistry & Cell Biology*, 568-584.

[6] Erices A, Conget P and Minguell JJ. (2000). Mesenchymal progenitor cells in human umbilical cord blood. *British Journal of Haematology*, 109, 235-242.

[7] Shetty P, Cooper K and Viwanathan C. (2010). Comparison of proliferative and multilineage differentiation potential of cord matrix, cord blood and bone marrow mesenchymal stem cells. *Asian J Transf Sci.*,4, 14-24.

[8] Kang TJ, Yeom J-E, Lee HJ et al. (2004). Growth kinetics of human mesenchymal stem cells from bone marrow and umbilical cord blood. *Acta Haematologica*,112, 230-233.

[9] Karen B, Susanne K, Herald K et al. (2004). Critical parameters for the isolation mesenchymal stem cells from umbilical cord blood. *Stem Cells*, 22, 625-634.

[10] Kolf C, Cho E and Tuan R. (2007). Mesenchymal stromal cells- Biology of adult mesenchymal stem cells: regulation of niche, self renewal and differentiation. *Arthritis Research and therapy*, 9, 204- 213.

[11] Simmons PJ and Torok-Storb B. (1991). Identification of stromal cell precursors in human bone marrow by a novel monoclonal antibody, STRO-1. *Blood*, 78, 55-62.

[12] Gronthos S, Zannettino AC, Hay SJ, et al. (2003). Molecular and cellular characterisation of highly purified stromal stem cells derived from human bone marrow. *J Cell Sci*, 116, 1827-1835.

[13] Dennis JE, Carbillet JP, Caplan AI, et al. (2002). The STRO-1+ marrow cell population is multipotential. *Cells Tissues Organs*, 170, 73-82.

[14] Bensidhoum M, Chapel A, Francois S, et al. (2004). Homing of *in vitro* expanded Stro-1^{-} or Stro-1^{+} human mesenchymal stem cells into the NOD/SCID mouse and their role in supporting human $CD34^{+}$ cell engraftment. *Blood*, 103:3313-3319.

[15] Carter RA and Wicks IP. (2001).Vascular cell adhesion molecule 1 (CD106): a multifaceted regulator of joint inflammation. *Arthritis Rheum*, 44, 985-994.

[16] M Dominici, K Le Blanc, I Mueller et al. (2006). Minimal criteria for defining Multipotent mesenchymal stromal cells: The International Society for cellular therapy position statement. *Cytotherapy* Vol. 8, No. 4, 315-317.

[17] Arnhold S, Heiduschka P, Klein H et al. (2006). Adenovirally transduced bone marrow stromal cells differentiate into pigment epithelial cells and induce rescue effects in RCS rats. *Invest Ophthalmol Vis Sci*, 47, 4121–4129.

[18] Arnhold S, Absenger Y, Klein H et al. (2007). Transplantation of bone marrow derived mesenchymal stem cells rescue photoreceptor cells in the dystrophic retina of the rhodopsin knockout mouse. *Graefes Arch Clin Exp Ophthalmol*, 245, 414–422.

[19] Nakagawa H, Akita S, Fukui M et al. (2005). Human mesenchymal stem cells successfully improve skin-substitute wound healing. *Br J Dermatol*, 153, 29 –36.

[20] Fu X, Fang L, Li X et al. (2006). Enhanced wound-healing quality with bone marrow mesenchymal stem cells autografting after skin injury. *Wound Repair Regen*, 14, 325–335.

[21] Morigi M, Imberti B, Zoja C et al. (2004). Mesenchymal stem cells are renotropic, helping to repair the kidney and improve function in acute renal failure. *J Am Soc Nephrol*, 15, 1794 –1804.

[22] Herrera MB, Bussolati B, Bruno S et al. (2004). Mesenchymal stem cells contribute to the renal repair of acute tubular epithelial injury. *Int J Mol Med*, 14, 1035–1041.
[23] D.G. Phinney and D.J Prockop. (2007). Mesenchymal stem cells: The state of transdifferentiation and modes of tissue repair- Current views. *Stem Cells*, 25, 2896-2902.
[24] Liechty KW, MacKenzie TC, Shaaban AF et al. (2000). Human mesenchymal stem cells engraft and demonstrate site-specific differentiation after in utero transplantation in sheep. *Nat Med*, 6, 1282-1286.
[25] Shetty P, Thakur A, Ravindran G, Viswanathan C. (2011). Directed therapeutic angiogenesis by mesenchymal stem cells from umbilical cord matrix in preclinical model of ischemic limb disease. *Stem Cell Studies*, 1, 97-104.
[26] Devine SM. (2002). Mesenchymal stem cells: Will they have a role in the clinic? *Journal of Cellular Biochemistry* Supplement, 38, 73-79.
[27] Bartholomew A, Sturgeon C, Siatskas M, et al. (2002). Mesenchymal stem cells suppress lymphocyte proliferation *in vitro* and prolong skin graft survival in vivo. *Exp Hematol*, 30(1), 42-8.
[28] Chabannes, D, Hill M, Merieau E, et al. (2007). A role for heme oxygenase-1 in the immunosuppressive effect of adult rat and human mesenchymal stem cells. *Blood*, 110(10), 3691-3694.
[29] Inoue, S, Popp FC, Koehl GE et al., (2006). Immunomodulatory Effects of Mesenchymal Stem Cells in a Rat Organ Transplant Model. *Transplantation*, 81(11), 1589-1595.
[30] Casiraghi, F, Azzollini N, Cassis P, et al., (2008). Pretransplant infusion of mesenchymal stem cells prolongs the survival of a semi allogeneic heart transplant through the generation of regulatory T cells. *J Immunol*, 181(6), 3933-46.
[31] Popp, F, Eggenhofer E, Renner P, et al., (2008). Mesenchymal stem cells can induce long-term acceptance of solid organ allografts in synergy with low-dose mycophenolate. *Transplant Immunology*, 20(1-2), 55-60.
[32] Zhou, H, Yi DH, Yu SQ, et al., (2006). Administration of Donor-Derived Mesenchymal Stem Cells Can Prolong the Survival of Rat Cardiac Allograft. *Transplantation Proceedings*, 38(9), 3046-3051.
[33] Tögel, F, Hu Z, Weiss K, et al. (2005). Administered mesenchymal stem cells protect against ischemic acute renal failure through differentiation-independent mechanisms. *American Journal of Physiology - Renal Physiology*, 289(1), F31-F42.

[34] Morigi, M., Introna M, Imberti B, et al. (2008). Human Bone Marrow Mesenchymal Stem Cells Accelerate Recovery of Acute Renal Injury and Prolong Survival in Mice. *Stem Cells*, 26(8), 2075-2082.

[35] Behr, L, Hekmati M, Lucchini A, et al. (2009). Evaluation of the effect of autologous mesenchymal stem cell injection in a large-animal model of bilateral kidney ischemia reperfusion injury. *Cell Prolif*,. 42(3), 284-297.

[36] Chamberlain G, Fox J, Ashton B, et al. (2007). Mesenchymal stem cells: their phenotype, differentiation capacity, immunological features and potential for homing. *Stem Cells*, 25, 2739–2749.

[37] Augello A, Tasso R, Negrini SM, et al. (2005). Bone marrow mesenchymal progenitor cells inhibit lymphocyte proliferation by activation of programmed death 1 pathway. *Eur J Immunol*, 35, 1482–1490.

[38] Sheng H, Wang Y, Jin Y, et al. (2008). A critical role of IFNγ priming MSC- mediated suppression of T cell proliferation through up regulation of B7-H1. *Cell Res*, 18, 846–857.

[39] Crisostomo, P, Troy M, Wang Y, et al. (2008). Surgically relevant aspects of stem cell paracrine effects. *Surgery*, 143(5), 577-581.

[40] Haynesworth, S.E., M.A. Baber, and A.I. Caplan. (1996). Cytokine expression by human marrow derived mesenchymal progenitor cells in vitro: effects of dexamethasone and IL-1 alpha. *J Cell Physiol*, 166(3), 585-592.

[41] Caplan, A.I. (2007). Adult mesenchymal stem cells for tissue engineering versus regenerative medicine. *J Cell Physiol*,. 213(2), 341-347.

[42] Chen, L, Tredget E, Wu P, et al. (2008). Paracrine factors of mesenchymal stem cells recruit macrophages and endothelial lineage cells and enhance wound healing. *PloS one*, 3(4), 1886.

[43] Corcione, A, Benvenuto F, Ferretti E, et al. (2006). Human mesenchymal stem cells modulate B-cell functions. *Blood*, 107(1), 367-372.

[44] Krampera, M, Glennie S, Dyson J, et al. (2003). Bone marrow mesenchymal stem cells inhibit the response of naive and memory antigen-specific T cells to their cognate peptide. *Blood*, 101, 3722-3729.

[45] Beyth, S, Borovsky Z, Mevorach D, et al. (2005). Human mesenchymal stem cells alter antigen-presenting cell maturation and induce T-cell unresponsiveness. *Blood*, 105(5), 2214-2219.

[46] Aggarwal, S and M.F. Pittenger. (2005). Human mesenchymal stem cells modulate allogeneic immune cell responses. *Blood*, 105(4), 1815-22.

[47] Meisel, R, Zibert A, Laryea M, et al.(2004). Human bone marrow stromal cells inhibit allogeneic T-cell responses by indoleamine 2,3-dioxygenase-mediated tryptophan degradation. *Blood*, 103(12), 4619-4621.

[48] Ren, G, Zhang L, Zhao X, et al. (2008). Mesenchymal stem cell-mediated immunosuppression occurs via concerted action of chemokines and nitric oxide. *Cell Stem Cell*, 2(2), 141-150.

[49] Nasef A, Mazurier C, Bouchet S, et al. (2008). Leukemia inhibitory factor: Role in human mesenchymal stem cells mediated immunosuppression. *Cellular Immunology*, 253(1-2), 16-22.

[50] Nasef A, Mathieu N, Chapel A, et al. (2007). Immunosuppressive Effects of Mesenchymal Stem Cells: Involvement of HLA-G. *Transplantation*, 84(2), 231-237.

[51] Selmani Z, Naji A, Gaiffe E, et al. (2009). HLA-G is a Crucial Immunosuppressive Molecule Secreted by Adult Human Mesenchymal Stem Cells. *Transplantation*, 87(Supplement), S62-S66.

[52] Doorn J, Moll G , Le Blanc K, et al. (2012). Therapeutic applications of mesenchymal stromal cells; paracrine effects and potential improvements. *Tissue Eng Part B Rev*. 2, 101-115

[53] Goshima J, Goldberg VM and Caplan AI. (1991). The origin of bone formed in composite grafts of porous calcium phosphate ceramic loaded with marrow cells. *Clin Orthop* 269, 274–283.

[54] Kadiyala S, Young RG, Thiede MA, et al. (1997). Culture expanded canine mesenchymal stem cells possess osteo-chondrogenic potential *in vivo* and *in vitro*. *Cell Transplant* 6, 125–134.

[55] Richards M, Huibregtse BA, Caplan AI, et al. (1999). Marrow-derived progenitor cell injections enhance new bone formation during distraction. *J Orthop Res* 17, 900–908.

[56] Johnstone B and Yoo JU. (1999). Autologous mesenchymal progenitor cells in articular cartilage repair. *Clin Orthop* 367, S156–S162.

[57] Young RG, Butler DL, Weber W, et al. (1998). Use of mesenchymal stem cells in a collagen matrix for Achilles tendon repair. *J Ortho Res* 16, 406–413.

[58] Koc ON, Gerson SL, Cooper BW, et al. (2000). Rapid hematopoietic recovery after co-infusion of autologous-blood stem cells and culture-

expanded marrow mesenchymal stem cells in advanced breast cancer patients receiving high-dose chemotherapy. *J Clin Oncol* 18, 307–316.
[59] Almeida-Porada G, Porada CD, Tran N, et al. (2000). Cotransplantation of human stromal cell progenitors into preimmune fetal sheep results in early appearance of human donor cells in circulation and boosts cell levels in bone marrow at later time points after transplantation. *Blood* 95, 3620–3627.
[60] Beauchamp JR, Morgan JE, Pagel CN, et al. (1999). Dynamics of myoblast transplantation reveal a discrete minority of precursors with stem cell-like properties as the myogenic source. *J Cell Biol* 144, 1113–1122.
[61] Gothot A, Loo JC, Clapp DW, et al. (1998). Cell cycle-related changes in repopulating capacity of human mobilized peripheral blood CD34 (+) cells in non-obese diabetic/severe combined immune deficient mice. *Blood* 92, 2641–2649.
[62] Lazarus HM, Haynesworth SE, Gerson SL, et al. (1995). *Ex vivo* expansion and subsequent infusion of human bone marrow derived stromal progenitor cells (mesenchymal progenitor cells): Implications for therapeutic use. *Bone Marrow Transplant* 16, 557–564.
[63] Gerson SL. (1999). Mesenchymal stem cells: No longer second class marrow citizens. *Nat Med* 5:262–264.
[64] Minguell J.J, Erices A and Conget P. (2001). Mesenchymal stem cells. *Exp Biol Med* Vol., 226(6), 507-520.
[65] Garcia-Olmo. (2009). Expanded adipose-derived stem cells for the treatment of complex perianal fistula: a phase II clinical trial. *Diseases of the colon and rectum*, 52, 79-86.
[66] Orlic D, Kajstura J, Chimenti S, et al. (2003). Bone marrow stem cells regenerate infarcted myocardium. *Pediatric transplantation*, 7 Suppl 3, 86-88.
[67] Zisa, D, Shabbir A, Suzuki G, et al. (2009). Vascular endothelial growth factor (VEGF) as a key therapeutic trophic factor in bone marrow mesenchymal stem cell-mediated cardiac repair. *Biochem Biophys Res Commun*, 390(3), 834-838.
[68] Nakamura T, Matsumoto K, Mizuno S, et al. (2005). Hepatocyte growth factor prevents tissue fibrosis, remodeling, anddysfunction in cardiomyopathic hamster hearts. *American Journal of Physiology - Heart and Circulatory Physiology*, 288(5), H2131-H2139.
[69] Shabbir A, Zisa D, Suzuki G, et al. (2009). Heart failure therapy mediated by the trophic activities of bone marrow mesenchymal stem

cells: a noninvasive therapeutic regimen. *Am J Physiol Heart Circ Physiol*, 296(6), 1888-1897.

[70] Menasche P. (2010). Cardiac cell therapy: Lessons from clinical trials. *Journal of Molecular and Cellular Cardiology*, 50(2), 258-265.

[71] Falanga V, Iwamoto S, Chartier M, et al. (2007). Autologous bone marrow-derived cultured mesenchymal stem cells delivered in a fibrin spray accelerate healing in murine and human cutaneous wounds. *Tissue engineering*, 13, 1299-1312.

[72] Suarez-Monteagudo C, Hernández-Ramírez P, Alvarez-González L, et al. (2009). Autologous bone marrow stem cell neurotransplantation in stroke patients. An open study. *Restorative Neurology and Neuroscience*, 27, 151-161.

[73] Venkataramana N.K., Kumar SK, Balaraju S, et al. (2010). Open-labeled study of unilateral autologous bone-marrow derived mesenchymal stem cell transplantation in Parkinson's disease. *Translational Research*, 155(2), 62-70.

[74] Karussis D, Karageorgiou C, Vaknin-Dembinsky A, et al. (2010). Safety and Immunological effects of Mesenchymal Stem Cell transplantation in patients with multiple sclerosis and amyotrophic lateral sclerosis. *Archives of Neurology*, 67(10), 1187-1194.

[75] Le Blanc K, Frassoni F, Ball L, et al. (2008). Mesenchymal stem cells for treatment of steroid-resistant, severe, acute graft-versus-host disease: a phase II study. The *Lancet*, 371(9624), 1579-1586.

[76] Le Blanc K, Rasmusson I, Sundberg B, et al. (2004). Treatment of severe acute graft-versus-host disease with third party haploidentical mesenchymal stem cells. Lancet, 363, 1439-1441.

[77] Caplan A.I, (2009). Why are MSCs therapeutic? New data: new insight. *J Pathol*, 217(2), 318-24.

[78] Tipnis S, Viswanathan C and Sen Majumdar A. (2010). Immunosuppressive properties of human umbilical cord-derived mesenchymal stem cells: role of B7-H1 and IDO. *Immunology and Cell Biology*, 88(8), 795-806.

[79] Barry FP and Murphy MM. (2004). Mesenchymal stem cells: clinical applications and biological characterization. *The International Journal of Biochemistry & Cell Biology*, 568-584.

[80] Shetty P, Ravindran G, Sarang S et al., (2009). Clinical grade mesenchymal stem cells transdifferentiated under xenofree conditions alleviates motor deficits in rat model of Parkinson's disease. *Cell Biology International*. 33 (8), 830-838.

[81] Shetty P, Bharucha K and Tanavde V. (2007). Human umbilical cord blood serum can replace fetal bovine serum in the culture of mesenchymal stem cells. *Cell Biology International*, 31, 293-298.

In: Cord Blood
Editor: Lisandra Vanostrand
ISBN: 978-1-62618-072-7

Chapter 3

Osteogenic Potential of Human Umbilical Cord-Derived Mesenchymal Stromal Cells

Kyoko Baba*[*]*, Yasuharu Yamazaki;
Akira Takeda and Eiju Uchinuma
Department of Plastic and Aesthetic Surgery, School of Medicine, Kitasato University, Minami-ku, Sagamihara, Kanagawa, Japan

Grants

Grant-in-Aid for Young Scientists (B) (21791750) and Grant-in-Aid for Scientific Research (B) (20592345), both from the Ministry of Education, Culture, Sports, Science and Technology, Japan

Abstract

The presence of umbilical cord-derived mesenchymal stem cells has been reported. In the present study, we used autoserum derived from the

[*] Correspondence should be addressed to: Kyoko Baba, MD, Department of Plastic and Aesthetic Surgery, School of Medicine, Kitasato University, 1-15-1 Kitasato, Minami-ku, Sagamihara, Kanagawa 252-0374, Japan, Phone number: +81-42-778-9074; facsimile number: +81-42-788-9327; e-mail address: kyokobaba@med.kitasato-u.ac.jp.

umbilical cord blood (UCB) of neonates in an attempt to examine the osteoblastic differentiation potential of umbilical cord-derived mesenchymal stromal cells (UC-MSCs) in nude mice.

UCB, hydroxyapatite, and rhBMP were used as the supply source of autologous serum, scaffold, and osteoinductive growth factor, respectively. MSCs, obtained from Wharton jelly and cultured for 3 to 4 weeks to induce their differentiation into osteoblasts, were implanted subcutaneously into the dorsum of male nude mice for 6 weeks before the assessment by real-time reverse transcriptase polymerase chain reaction of osteoblast marker expression.

UCB-derived autologous serum was sufficient for the culture and implantation of UC-MSCs. The osteoblastic differentiation potential of UC-MSCs was demonstrated in nude mice by the conduct of immunohistochemical staining and by the investigation of osteoblast marker expression. Our results suggest the osteogenic potential of UC-MSCs and provide basic evidence for the realization of regenerative medicine using materials obtained from UC and UCB.

Keywords: Regenerative medicine; Human umbilical cord blood; Mesenchymal stromal cell; Osteogenesis; Autologous tissue; Fibrin

1. Introduction

The usefulness of mesenchymal stromal cells (MSCs) in regenerative medicine is becoming widely recognized. Mesenchymal stem cells are fully established as essential materials for regenerative medicine and are found in many tissues, e.g., bone marrow and adipose tissue. Among them, bone marrow is the most common supply source of mesenchymal stem cells for osteogenesis. In recent years, the clinical applications of bone marrow-derived mesenchymal stem cells (BM-MSCs) in the field of craniomaxillofacial surgery have been sporadically reported [1, 2]. On the other hand, recent studies [3, 4, 5] revealed the presence of mesenchymal stem cells in sorts of tissues. The umbilical cord (UC) is also one of tissues where mesenchymal stem cells are present. In general, concerns about medical safety (e.g., immune response to biomedical materials, infection, and adverse events) and ethical issues about the source of biomedical materials arise when applying regenerative medicine to the clinical settings. Since the use of autologous tissue can minimize many of these issues that originate from the use of allogenic or xenogenic tissue, we consider that autologous tissue is preferred biomedical material for clinical use in regenerative medicine. UC, whose abundant tissue volume is noninvasively available from the neonate at birth, has good clinical applicability to the patient him/herself if allowed to be used as autologous tissue that causes less ethical, medical, and safety issues. In recent years, diagnostic echography of fetuses has revealed congenital anomalies involving deficits in maxillofacial bones. Consequently, the number of pregnant women visiting our department for the prenatal consultation of their fetus diagnosed with alveolar cleft has increased. The renatal diagnosis of congenital craniofacial anomalies allowed successful preparation for the collection at the time of birth. Therefore, we focused on UC as the supply source of autologous osteogenic cells.

Osteogenesis in a bone defect at the site of alveolar cleft is important for patients with cleft lip and palate to obtain dental articulation. In accordance with a published study [6], we have conducted gingivoperiostealplasty when required during cheiloplasty and have prepared the ground for osteogenesis. However, some pediatric patients have presented difficulty undergoing orthodontic treatment in their schoolage or later because of the insufficient volume of formed bone tissue. In addition, because of the grafted bone absorption and bone growth, repeated operations are often required, which imposes a heavy burden on the pediatric patients. Hence, with intention for diminution of surgical suffering, we have investigated osteogenesis by regenerative medicine at the site of bone defect in these patients.

In the present study, we intended to maximally purvey materials for regenerative medicine with autologous tissues. Namely, we used UC-derived mesenchymal stromal cells (UC-MSCs) and UC blood (UCB)-derived autoserum to examine the cytobiological features of UC-MSCs *in vitro*. Furthermore, we investigated the osteoblastic differentiation potential of UC-MSCs *in vivo*. In addition, as a preliminary study, we investigate structure of umbilical cord blood-derived fibrin (UCB-fibrin) as scaffold.

2. Materials and Methods

With the approval by the ethics committee at Kitasato University, the present study was conducted after having obtained written informed consent from all pregnant women. UC and UCB collected from neonates, who had not presented any problem during pregnancy and delivery and who had been born at term, were used.

2.1. Treatment of UCB

UCB was collected by puncturing the umbilical vein after the expulsion of the placenta. Immediately after collection, UCB was mixed with ACD-A (Terumo Co., Ltd., Tokyo, Japan) at a volume ratio of 1:1 to perform anticoagulation. Subsequently, the mixture was centrifuged twice (2,400 rpm, 10 min; 3,600 rpm, 10 min) at 20°C to obtain UCB platelet-rich plasma (UCB-PRP) and platelet-poor plasma(UCB-PPP). Serum was obtained from this UC-derived plasma before use in the culture of MSCs. PRP was cryopreserved at -80°C until immediately before use and was used at the time of implantation into nude mice.

2.2. Pretreatment of UC

After the collection of UCB, UC was cut into about 10-cm sections and was washed with phosphate buffered saline (PBS; Wako Pure Chemical Industries Co., Ltd., Osaka, Japan) up to the moment when no attached blood remained. The umbilical arteries, the umbilical vein, and Wharton jelly (WJ) other than the periumbilical membrane were cut into about 5-mm sections. In accordance with published modified methods [7, 8], these sections were incubated by using Dulbecco's modified eagle's medium (DMEM) added with 10% autoserum derived from UCB in the 25-cm^2 flask (Sumitomo Bakelite Co., Ltd., Tokyo, Japan) under the conditions of 5% CO_2 and 37°C. Media were replaced for the first time at 1 week after the onset of the culture and every 3 days thereafter. Following the emergence of adhesive spindle-shaped cells, the WJ sections were removed at about 2 weeks after the onset of the culture. The culture was continued until the moment when cells became subconfluent (Figure 1).

2.3. Assessment of the Osteoblastic- and Adipogenic Differentiation Potential of UC-Mscs

The differentiation of UC-MSCs into osteoblasts and adipose cells was attempted to assess the osteoblastic- and adipogenic differentiation potential of WJ-derived cells.

One portion of subconfluent primary cultured cells was induced for differentiation into osteoblasts by changing the medium to the NH OsteoDiff

Medium, while the other portion was induced for differentiation into adipose cells by changing the medium to NH AdipoDiff Medium (Miltenyi Biotec GmbH, Bergisch Gladbach, Germany). These portions of cells were stained with alizarin red and oil red, respectively, before observation with a stereoscopic microscope.

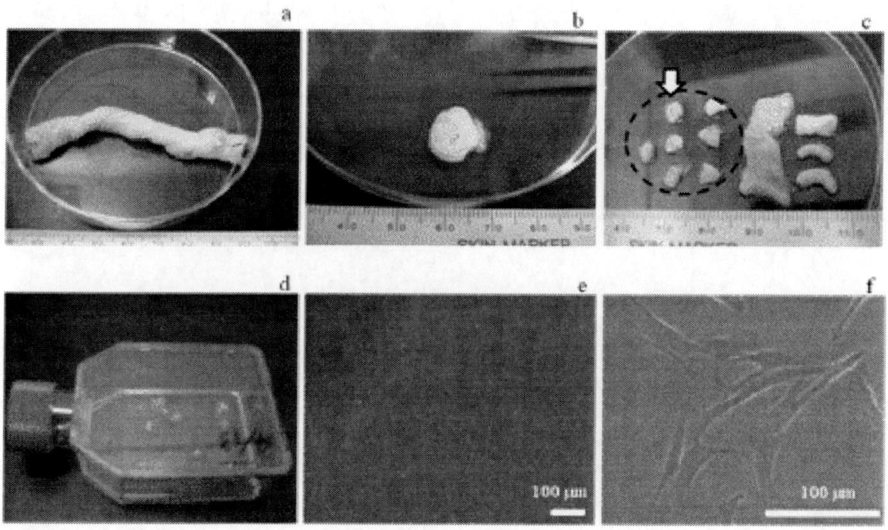

Figure 1. Pretreatment of the umbilical cord. The umbilical cord was collected after the expulsion of the placenta.

a. The umbilical cord was cut into about 10-cm sections and was washed with phosphate buffered saline up to the moment when no attached blood remained.

b. Cross section of the umbilical cord. The umbilical cord was washed up to the moment when no attached blood remained also in the vascular lumen. The cross section identified the umbilical vein and arteries.

c. After the removal of the periumbilical membrane, umbilical arteries, and umbilical vein, Wharton jelly was cut into about 5-mm sections (white arrow).

d. Wharton jelly was cultured in Dulbecco's modified eagle's medium added with 10% autoserum.

e. Outgrowth cells from Wharton jelly that were observed at 2 weeks after the onset of the culture.

f. Outgrowth cells were adhesive spindle-shaped cells.

2.4. Seeding of UC-MSCs to Hydroxyapatite(HA) and Implantation Thereof into Nude Mice

In accordance with a published study [9], the HA [$Ca_{10}(PO_4)_6(OH)_2$; Pentax Corporation, Tokyo, Japan] disks of 5 mm in diameter and of 2 mm in thickness with a porosity of 85% (pore diameter: 100 to 500 μm) were used. The seeding of primary cultured cells (1×10^5 cells/disk) was performed, and DMEM was used to conduct 1-week culture to wait for cell infiltration into HA. Subsequently, the medium was changed to NH OsteoDiff Medium in which 300 ng/mL rhBMP had been added (Miltenyi Biotech) to conduct 3-week culture. Samples were subcutaneously implanted into the dorsum of male nude mice BALB/Ca Jcl-nu nu/nu (Clea Japan, Inc., Tokyo, Japan) and were removed at 6 weeks later.

2.5. Histological and Immunohistochemical Assessments

Specimens removed from mice were fixed with 10% formalin, followed by decalcification with KCX (Falma Co., Ltd., Tokyo, Japan). After washing, the decalcified samples were embedded in paraffin, cut to about 3-μm sections, stained with HE, and observed with an optical microscope. Immunohistochemical staining followed published procedures [10]. Namely, specimens were stained with the anti-human osteocalcin (OC) antibody and the anti-human mitochondrial antibody before assessment with a fluorescence microscope.

2.6. Assessment of the Expression of Osteoblast Markers

In accordance with published procedures [11], RNeasy MiniKit (Qiagen, Valencia, CA) was used to extract total RNA in HA that had been removed from nude mice according to this protocol; cDNA was thus prepared. Real-time reverse transcriptase-polymerase chain reaction (RT-PCR) was performed to assess the expressions of human osteoblast markers, runt-related gene 2 (Runx2), alkaline phosphatase (ALP), and OC after hybridization. On the other hand, specimens *in vitro*, which had not been induced for differentiation (control), were also assessed with the same markers. Five specimens each were used to determine the expression of the markers, and both categories of the specimens were compared according to unpaired

Student's t-test. A value of < 0.05 was considered statistically significant. The PCR primer sequences for Runx2, ALP, and OC were designed based on the Primer 3 GeneBank sequence, and the PCR primers were designed using the Primer 3 software program (http://primer3.sourceforge.net/). The primer sequences were as follows: for RUNX2, I-F: ttcaggtgcttcagaactgg and I-R: gactggcggggtgtaagtaa; for ALP, I-F: gtacgagctgaacaggaacaacg and I-R: cttggcttttccttcatggtg; and for OC, I-F: gactgtgacgagttggctga and I-R: agcagagcgacaccctagac.

2.7. Assessment of UCB-Derived Fibrin Net Structure

A catalyst, in which calcium chloride was added to UCB-derived thrombin at a volume ratio of 3:1, was added to UCB-PPP at a volume ratio of 10:1 in order to precipitate fibrin. UCB-fibrin and UCB-PRP were cryopreserved at -80°C up to the time of use. These were thawed at room temperature just before use. The structure of thawed UCB-fibrin was examined by scanning electron microscopy (SEM; Vacc. 5kV, S-4500 FE Type, Hitachi Ltd. JAPAN).

UCB-fibrin, which was cut into pieces of 5 mm in size, was put into the flask, and primary outgrowth cells were seeded (1×10^5 cells/piece). DMEM was used to conduct 1-week culture to wait for cell infiltration into UCB-fibrin. Afterwards, the medium was changed to NH OsteoDiff Medium, and this medium was used for differentiation induction to osteoblasts during 3 weeks. When the medium was changed to NH OsteoDiff Medium, UCB-PRP was added to the medium at the ratio of 300 nL/mL only at the first time. UCB-fibrin seeded with UC-MSCs was also examined by scanning electron microscopy.

3. Results

3.1. Volume of Autoserum Derived from UCB

The volume of UCB collected from 17 samples was measured and ranged between 27 mL and 74 mL, with an average volume of 50 mL. The volume of serum collected from UCB ranged between 11 mL and 44 mL, with an average volume of 22 mL. In the present study, the actual volume of serum required to culture 1 × 10^5 cells from primary culture to implantation into nude mice ranged between 3.6 mL and 4.2 mL.

3.2. Assessment of the Osteoblastic- and Adipogenic Differentiation Potential of Cells *In Vitro*

The samples of UC-MSC—which had been induced to differentiation into osteoblasts—were stained extracellularly and diffusely with alizarin red, verifying the presence of calcium. Furthermore, UC-MSCs—which had been induced to differentiation into adipose cells—showed intracellular lipid droplets that were stained with oil red (Figure 2).

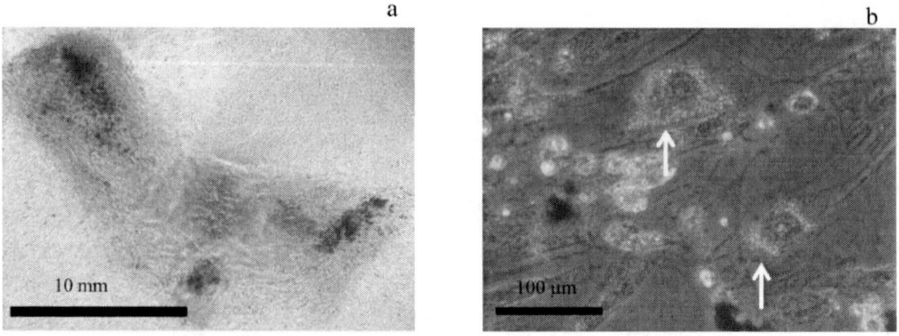

Figure 2. *In vitro* assessment of the osteoblastic- and adipogenic differentiation potential of umbilical cord-derived mesenchymal stromal cells. Umbilical cord-derived mesenchymal stromal cells (UC-MSCs) were induced to differentiate into osteoblasts and adipose cells.

a) Staining with alizarin red - The samples of UC-MSCs, which had been induced to differentiation into osteoblasts, were stained extracellularly and diffusely with alizarin red.

b) Staining with oil red - The samples of UC-MSCs, which had been induced to differentiation into adipose cells, showed intracellular lipid droplets that were stained with oil red (white arrows).

3.3. Immunohistochemical Assessments

The formation of immature bone tissue was occasionally found in the pores of the HA disks. In immunohistochemical staining, the portions confirmed by HE stain to contain bone tissue were positive for both the human anti-OC antibody and the anti-human mitochondrial antibody. These facts verified that cells in the relevant portions produced OC and originated from humans, demonstrating the successful osteoblastic differentiation of UC-MSCs *in vivo* (Figure 3).

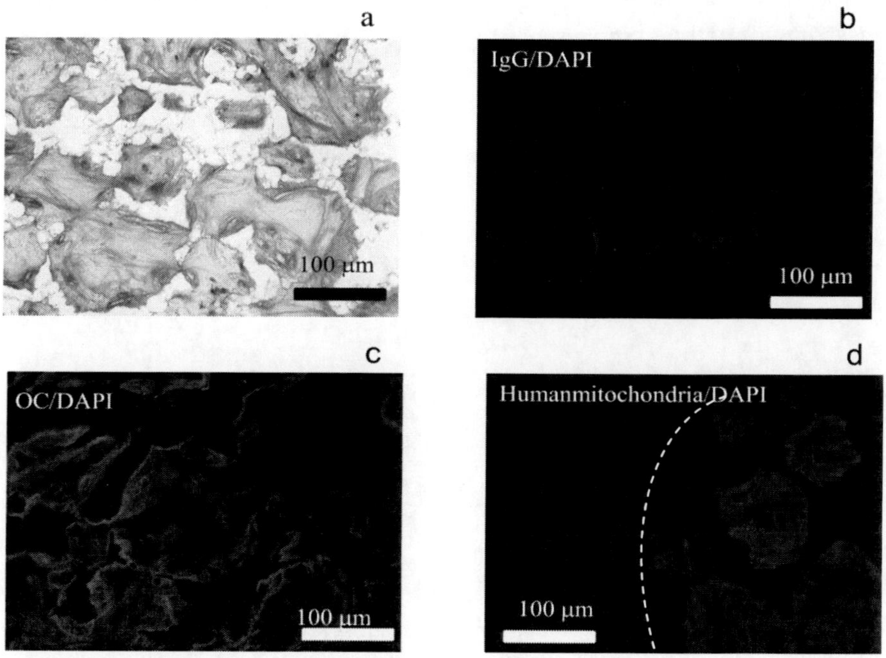

Figure 3. Histological and immunohistochemical staining of specimens from nude mice

a) H&E stain: immature bone tissue is found in the pores of the hydroxyapatite (HA) disks.

b) Immunohistochemical staining. Negative control: desorption atmospheric pressure photoionization.

c) Immunohistochemical staining: The interior of the HA disks was stained with the anti-human osteocalcin antibody.

d) Immunohistochemical staining: The interior of the HA disk pores was stained with the anti-human mitochondrial antibody. The dotted line indicates the HA border. The left and right sides of the dotted line in the figure represent murine tissue outside HA and human-derived cells implanted into the interior of HA, respectively. IgG, immunoglobulin G; DAPI, 4',6-diamidino-2-phenylindole; and OC, osteocalcin.

3.4. Expression of Osteoblast Markers by real-time RT-PCR

Specimens *in vivo* showed high values of Runx2 and ALP as compared with undifferentiated UC-MSCs, and exhibited significant differences (P < 0.05) according to unpaired Student's t-test (Figure 4). OC markers had high values of OC without showing a significant difference against control and suggested the osteoblastic differentiation potential of UC-MSCs.

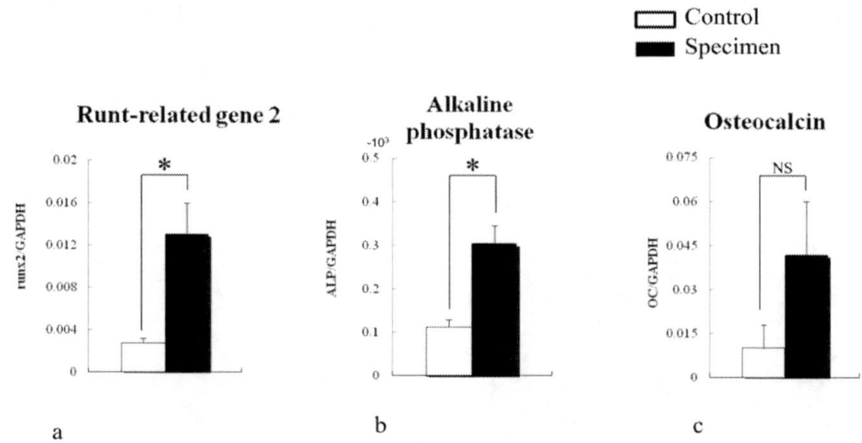

Figure 4. Expressions of osteoblast markers by real-time reverse transcriptase-polymerase chain reaction. Unpaired Student's t-test was performed to make statistical analyses. Consequently, Runx2 and alkaline phosphatase showed significant differences (*P < 0.05) (a and b), while osteocalcin did not (c).

3.5. Structure of UCB-Derived Fibrin Net

UCB-derived fibrin net of about 4 to 6 cm^3 was formed per UCB of about 40 mL. SEM revealed the reticulated structure of thawed fibrin in which fibrin fibers were intertangled. This three-dimensional structure was relatively homogeneous in both the superficial and deep layers (Figure 5). This structure was present continuously from areas near the surface to deeper areas. A thawed fibrin exhibited numbers of spindle-shaped cells and granular materials. These autologous UC-MSCs naturally infiltrated into UCB-fibrin only by seeding.

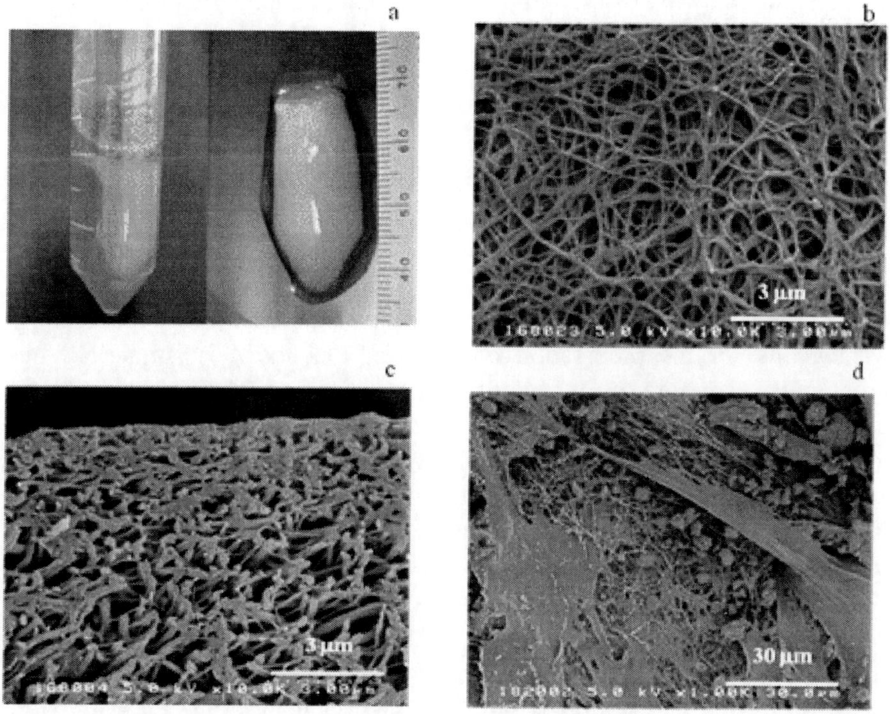

Figure 5. Umbilical cord blood-derived fibrin (UCB-fibrin) immediately after thawing

a) Macroscopic appearance

b) Scanning electron microscopy image (SEM) of the UCB-fibrin surface showing a reticular structure

c) SEM image of the UCB-fibrin cross section showing a reticular structure that is preserved to deep layers

d) SEM image of the UCB-fibrin cross section showing spindle-shaped cells and granular materials in its interior.

4. Discussion

In preclinical studies, fetal bovine serum (FBS) is commonly used to culture cells. When considering the preparation of hybrid-type bone substitute that is applicable clinically, however, FBS involves various medical issues, e.g., immune response induced by remaining bovine serum proteins, possible presence of unknown viruses, and potential contamination with prions. Serum-free media for mesenchymal stem cells have also been developed as countermeasures for these problems of FBS. However, the long-term safety of all components that serum-free media contain still remains to be established. In consideration of these issues and ethical aspects, the use of autoserum is ideal. Media using autoserum have been reported not to be inferior in quality to media using FBS when preparing a hybrid-type bone substitute by using human bone marrow-derived mesenchymal stem cells [8]. Furthermore, the involvement of serum proteins at the time of adhesion between osteoblasts and HA has been suggested [12, 13], leading us to consider that the use of serum is advantageous for the preparation of a hybrid-type bone substitute. In the present study, therefore, we intended to use autoserum in order to culture UC-MSCs by using UCB as its supply source. The collection of UCB is noninvasive to the fetus, and the collection procedure is easy to perform because the umbilical vein is punctured after the expulsion of the placenta. Furthermore, the average collection volume is 50 mL, being abundant as blood to be collected from the fetus. The volume of serum obtained from UCB was 22 mL on average. Therefore, a sufficient volume of autoserum could be obtained from UCB for the culture of 1×10^5 cells as required by the present study protocol. UCB-derived autoserum noninvasively obtained in abundance was useful for the preparation of a hybrid-type bone substitute by using UC-MSCs and HA.

The portions confirmed by HE stain to contain bone tissue were immunohistochemically stained with both the anti-OC antibody and the anti-human mitochondrial antibody, which verified that OC-producing cells had been derived from humans. Real-time RT-PCR revealed the expression of osteoblast markers (Runx2 and ALP), which confirmed the cellular activity of osteoblasts. Osteoblasts exhibited differences in marker expression according to their differentiation stage. The osteoblast markers are expressed according to differentiation stage in order of Runx2, ALP, and OC (14) (15). Differences in marker expression were considered attributable to differences in cell differentiation stage. Cells measured were considered to be found at the early stage of differentiation.

Cell, scaffold, and growth factor are required for regenerative medicine. UC-MSCs used differentiated into osteoblasts and adipose cells *in vitro*, thus verifying their osteoblastic- and adipogenic differentiation potential. rhBMP was used as an osteoinductive factor at the time of differentiation induction. UCB-PRP was implanted together with the sample for the purpose of enhancing neovascularization from the implantation bed to the sample and of assisting osteogenesis. HA used as the scaffold had already been recognized as a useful scaffold for osteogenesis [16, 17, 18]. Recent studies [19-22] have indicated that a three-dimensional scaffold is advantageous for the differentiation of mesenchymal cells. Furthermore, a group of researchers [23] reported that neovascularization *in vivo* is affected by the porosity and pore diameter of the HA disks. The pores of the HA disks had a three-dimensional structure, and not only cell infiltration but also neovascularization was found in the pores; however, formed bone tissue was immature. We conjecture the following three conceivable causes for this observation: 1) the number of osteogenic cells that had been seeded resulted to be insufficient; 2) the subcutis—where no bone tissue is formed naturally—was used as the graft bed, leading to afford an environment that was unideal for osteogenesis. Nevertheless, a group of investigators [8] successfully obtained mature bone tissue by using BM-MSCs according the subcutaneous implantation procedure. Furthermore, osseous healing was comparable in an animal study where adipose-, periosteum-, and bone marrow-derived mesenchymal stem cells had been implanted into a bone deficit [24]; and 3) MSCs included in UC-MSCs were probably more primordial. Therefore, a further induction may be required to differentiate UC-MSCs into osteoblasts. Another group of researchers [25] described that cells have an intrinsically limited life span, making it difficult to proliferate cells unlimitedly. UC is a tissue that is fated to perish in about 10 months. Therefore, it is possible that UC presents a life span shorter than that of other cells and also has different tolerability against the life span. Our study provided positive evidence for osteogenesis by culturing UC-MSCs with UCB-derived autoserum and by using HA as the scaffold. UC-MSCs were thus suggested to be a potential material for regenerative medicine. On the other hand, we consider it necessary to further investigate safety concerns, e.g., cell canceration, prior to the clinical application of UC-MSCs.

In recent years, the differentiation of MSCs has been indicated to require three-dimensional culture [19-22]. The structure of thawed UCB-fibrin resembled that from peripheral blood of adults, in which fiber components were intertangled homogeneously. The fibrin net has a reticular structure in which fibers are intertwined intricately and constant spaces are present among fibers. Therefore, we consider that the fibrin net provides an environment which allows cellular infiltration and can contribute to the three dimensional structure. Also in the present study, autologous UC-MSCs naturally infiltrated into UCB-fibrin only by seeding.SEM verified that the fibrin structure preserved its three-dimensionality to deep layers without any artificial manipulation, leading us to consider that the structure complies with the culture of MSCs. Furthermore, we deem that the fibrin net has excellent cytophillicity because it is derived from autologous tissues and is a physiological substance which appears at the time of wound healing.

Conclusion

We used noninvasively obtained autologous tissues and a biomaterial already in clinical use to successfully verify their potential of allowing bone regenerative medicine. Furthermore, we examined the osteoblastic differentiation potential of UC-MSCs by using MSCs supplied from UC, growth factor and serum for cell culture purveyed from UCB, and HA as the scaffold; immature bone tissue was thus obtained. These results provide basic evidence for the realization of regenerative medicine using autologous tissues derived from patients with cleft lip and palate. In the future, we will intend to investigate the research strategies and technical procedures in an attempt to obtain safer hybrid-type artificial bone for clinical application. SEM verified that the fibrin structure preserved its three-dimensionality to deep layers without any artificial manipulation, leading us to consider that the structure complies with the culture of MSCs.

Acknowledgments

The present study received Grant-in-Aid for Young Scientists (B) (21791750) and Grant-in-Aid for Scientific Research (B) (20592345), both from the Ministry of Education, Culture, Sports, Science and Technology, Japan.

References

[1] Wongchuensoontorn C, Liebehenschel N, Schwarz U, Schmelzeisen R, Gutwald R, Ellis E, Sauerbier S.: Application of a new chair-side method for the harvest of mesenchymal stem cells in a patient with nonunion of a fracture of the atrophic mandible – A case report. *J Craniomaxillofac Surg* 37: 155 161, 2009.

[2] Behnia H, Khojasteh A, Soleimani M, Tehranchi A, Atashi A: Repair of alveolar cleft defect with mesenchymal stem cells and platelet derived growth factors: A preliminary report. *J Craniomaxillofac Surg* 40: 2 7, 2012.

[3] Sarugaser R, Lickorish D, Baksh D, Hosseini MM, Davies JE: Human umbilical cord perivascular (HUCPV) cells: A source of mesenchymal progenitors. *Stem cells* 23: 220 209, 2005.

[4] Kern S, Eichler H, Stoeve J, Bieback K: Comparative analysis of mesenchymal stem cells from bone marrow, umbilical cord blood or adipose tissue. *Stem cells* 24: 1294 1301, 2006.

[5] Pivorinūas A, Bernotiene E, Unguryte A, Valiuniene S, Drasutiene G, Venalis A: Isolation and differentiation of mesenchymal stem-like cells from human umbilical cord vein endothelium and subendothelium. *Biologija* 2: 99 103, 2006.

[6] Millard DR, Latham RA, Huifen X, Spiro S, Morovic C: Cleft lip and palate treated by presurgical orthopedics, gingivoperiosteoplasty, and lip adhesion (POPLA) compared with previous lip adhesion method: a preliminary study of serial dental casts. *Plast Reconstr Sur* 103: 1630 1644, 1999.

[7] Okamoto K, Miyoshi S, Toyoda M, Hida N, Ikegam Y, Makino H, Nishiyama N, Tsuji H, Cui CH, Segawa K, Uyama T, Kami D, Matsumoto K, Saito H, Yoshimura Y, Ogawa S, Aeba R, Yozu R, Umezawa A: Working cardiomyocytes exhibiting plateau action potentials from human placenta-derived extraembryonic mesodermal cells. *Exp Cell Res* 313: 2550 2562, 2007.

[8] MatsuoA, Yamazaki Y, Takase C, Aoyagi K, Uchinuma E: Osteogenic potential of human bone marrow-derived mesenchymal stem cells cultured with autologous serum. *J Craniofac Surg* 19: 693 700, 2008.

[9] Takase C, Yamazaki Y, Matsuo A, Aoyagi K, Takeda A, Uchinuma E: Differing effects of allogenic heterologous sera and scaffold structures on the bone forming ability of undifferentiated mesenchymal cells. *The Kitasato Med J* 40: 122 128, 2010.

[10] Abe S, Yamaguchi S, Watanabe A, Hamada K, Amagasa T: Hard tissue regeneration capacity of apical derived cells (APDCs) from human tooth with immature apex. *Biochem Biophys Res Commun* 371: 90 93, 2008.

[11] Ogata S, Ogihara Y, Nomoto K, Akiyama K, Nakahata Y, Sato K, Minoura K, Kokubo K, Kobayashi H, Ishii M: Clinical score and transcript abundance patterns identify Kawasaki disease patients who

may benefit from addition of methylprednisolone. *Pediat Res* 19: 577 584, 2009.

[12] Yamamoto N, Isobe M, Negishi A, Yoshimasu H, Shimokawa H, Ohya K, Amagasa T, Kasugai S: Effects of autologous serum on osteoblastic differentiation in human bone marrow cells. *J Med Dent Sci* 50: 63 69, 2003.

[13] Okamoto M, Dohi Y, Ohgushi H, Shimaoka H, Ikeuchi M, Matsushima A, Yonemasu K, Hosoi H: Osteogenic potential of human influence of the porosity of hydroxyapatite ceramics on in vitro and in vivo bone formation by cultured rat bone marrow stromal cells. *J Mater Sci Mater Med* 17: 327 336, 2006

[14] Sun H, Ye F, Wan J, Shi Y, Tu Z, Bao J, Qin M, Bu H, Li Y: The upregulation of osteoblast marker genes in mesenchymal stem cells prove the osteoinductivity of hydroxyapatite/tricalcium phosphate biomaterial. *Transplantation* 40: 2645 2648, 2008.

[15] Meister G, Tuschl T: Mechanisms of gene silencing by double-stranded RNA. *Nature* 431: 343 349, 2004.

[16] Ohgushi H, Okumura M, Yoshikawa T, Inboue K, Senpuku N, Tamai S, Shors EC: Bone formation process in porous calcium carbonate and hydroxyapatite. *J Biomed Mater Res* 26: 885 895, 1992.

[17] Okumura M, Ohgushi H, Dohi Y, Katuda T, Tamai S, Koerten HK, Tabata S: Osteoblastic phenotype expression on the surface of hydroxyapatite ceramics. *J Biomed Mater Res* 37: 122 129, 1997.

[18] Ohgushi H, Kitamura S, Kotobuki N, Hirose M, Machida H, Muraki K, Takakura Y: Clinical application of marrow mesenchymal stem cells for hard tissue repair. *Yonsei Med* J 45:61 67, 2004.

[19] Schneider RK, Puellen A, Kramann R, Raupach K, Bornemann J, Knuechel R, Perez-Bouza A, Neuss S: The osteogenic differentiation of adult bone marrow and perinatal umbilical mesenchymal stem cells and matrix remodeling in three-dimensional collagen scaffolds. *Biomaterials* 31: 467 480, 2010.

[20] McMahon LA, Reid AJ, Campbell VA, Prendergast PJ: Regulatory effects of mechanical strain on the chondrogenic differentiation of MSCs in a collagen-GAG scaffold: Experimental and computational analysis. *Anal Biomed Eng* 36: 185 194, 2008.

[21] Moisenovich MM, Pustovalova OL, Arhipova AY, Vasiljeva TV, Sokolova OS, Bogush VG, Debabov VG, Sevastianov VI, Kirpichnikov MP, Agapov II. *In vitro* and *in vivo* biocompatibility studies of a

recombinant analogue of spidroin 1 scaffolds. *J Biomed Mater Res A* 96: 125 131, 2011.

[22] Lee J, Cuddihy MJ, Kotov NA: Three-dimensional cell culture matrices: State of the art. *Tissue Eng Part B Rev* 14: 61 86, 2008.

[23] Nishikawa M, Myoui A, Ohgushi H, Ikeuchi M, Tamai N, Yoshikawa H: Bone tissue engineering using novel interconnected porous hydroxyapatite ceramics combined with marrow mesenchymal cells: quantitative and three-dimensional image analysis. *Cell Transplant* 13: 367 376, 2044.

[24] Stockmann P, Park J, von Wilmowsky C, Nkenke E, Felszeghy E, Dehner JF, Schmitt C, Tudor C, Schlegel KA: Guided bone regeneration in pig calvarial bone defects using autologous mesenchymal stem/progenitor cells—A comparison of different tissue sources. *J Craniomaxillofac Surg*, in press, 2011.

[25] Terai M, Uyama T, Sugiki T, Li XY, Umezawa A, Kiyono T: Immortalization of human fetal cells: The life span of umbilical cord blood-derived cells can be prolonged without manipulating $p16^{INK4a}$/RB braking pathway. *Mol Cell Biol* 16: 1491 1499, 2005.

In: Cord Blood
Editor: Lisandra Vanostrand

ISBN: 978-1-62618-072-7

Chapter 4

Public *versus* Private Cord Blood Banking: Ethical Implications

Elena Salvaterra[*]
Unit of Bioethics, Scientific Institute IRCCS "Medea",
Associazione La Nostra Famiglia, Lecco, Italy

To Leo Jonathan,
my loved son

Abstract

This chapter seeks to identify some ethical issues associated with public and private cord blood banks. After a brief report on existing cord blood banks worldwide, it aims to stimulate ethical reflections about allogenic versus autologous cord blood transplants. Whereas allogenic (related and unrelated) transplantation of umbilical cord blood is scientifically recognized as a proven treatment for several diseases affecting both children and adults, private cord blood banks promote a service – namely, the storage of the newborn cord blood for autologous transplant – which is not presently supported by clinical evidence. This

[*] Correspondence author: Elena Salvaterra, JD, PhD, Unit of Bioethics, Scientific Institute IRCCS "Medea", Associazione La Nostra Famiglia, Via D. Luigi Monza, 20, 23842, Lecco, Italy, msalvaterra@bp.lnf.it , elenasalvaterra@yahoo.com.

raises critical issues in ethical terms ranging from the legitimacy of the informed consent process to the breach of the principle of justice requiring a fair distribution of available cord blood units among patients who need a cord blood transplant.

Introduction

Since the first umbilical cord blood transplant (UCBT), performed in 1988 for the treatment of a child affected by Franconi Anemia, surprising steps have been made into the hematopoietic stem cell transplantation and new challenges opened, particularly associated with the potential of non-hematopoietic cord blood cells [1].

Cord blood transplant (CBT) is, nowadays, a standard treatment option in pediatric transplantation and it is an increasingly recognized as a hematopoietic stem cell source for adults [2, 3].

Evidence that long-term survival after cord blood transplant (CBT) for both children and adults is comparable to that of bone marrow transplantation (BMT) makes the increasing utilization of cord blood transplant and banking likely [4-7].

Moreover, the greater histocompatibility of cord blood transplants relative to BMT extends cord blood transplantation access to racial and ethnic minorities, who are still underrepresented on donor registries worldwide [8].

A crucial factor that has helped to make umbilical cord blood transplants a successful treatment for bone marrow disorders, both genetic and acquired [9], has been the development of public not-for-profit cord blood banks. Since the first CBT, an increasing number of public cord blood banks have been established worldwide to collect and store cord blood for allogenic (related or unrelated) transplantation [10]

Today, there are more than 100 active public cord blood banks, mostly based in Europe, the Middle East, North- and South America, and Australia [11]. Moreover, a number of networks including Netcord (http://www. netcord.org), Asiacord (http://asiacord.org), and Bone Marrow Donors Worldwide (http://bmdw.org), have been developed with an estimated inventory of 600,000 cord blood units banked and more than 20,000 cord blood units distributed worldwide [10].

At the same time, private, for-profit cord blood banks have been established to collect and store the newborn child cord blood for personal use. Today, nearly 150 private cord blood banks are listed on the "Parent's Guide to Cord Blood" website (http://parentsguidecordblood.org/) most notably in the USA, Europe, Central and South America and more recently Australia, New Zealand, the Middle East, India and other parts of Asia [12].

Private, for-profit cord blood banks – also known as commercial cord blood banks – offer to store, for a variable fee, the cord blood of the newborn in view of a future, possible autologous transplantation. Over the last 15 years, about 900,000 cord blood units have been stored privately for personal use, and about 100 autologous transplants have been performed worldwide [13].

The explosion of private cord blood banks has been and still remains controversial from both scientific and ethical perspectives. What makes private cord blood banks problematic is the fact that they offer a service – actually, the potentially unlimited storage of the newborn cord blood for personal use - not supported by clinical evidence [12-14].

Medical organizations [9, 15-17], ethical commissions [18] and policy makers [19] have evoked the lack of proven data supporting the use of newborn cord blood and autologous transplantations.

In spite of this, private cord blood banking remains a desirable chance for many parents willing to guarantee a "biological insurance" [12] to their children.

Based on this scenario, this chapter aims to identify some ethical implications associated with public cord blood banks *versus* private cord blood banks.

The first implication is about the consent given by expectant parents to privately store the cord blood of their newborn child.

According to the ethical principles governing the biomedical practice [20-21], the parents' informed consent to store the newborn cord blood for personal use is valid when given by subjects competent to consent to, freely express their choice and be truthfully informed on the available options.

Based on recent studies, private cord blood banks often provide expectant parents with inadequate information, because they promise clinical outcomes that are not well proven at present [12]. As a consequence, the consent given by expectant parents is not fully compliant according to the required ethical principles, which must give potential decision makers complete and truthful information.

The second ethical implication associated with commercial cord blood banks pertains to the limited access to cord blood transplants derived from the storage of newborn cord blood for personal use. Public cord blood banks contribute, at least in part, to expand the donor registries worldwide, permitting more patients to find a suitable match thanks to the increasing number of cord blood units made available for allogenic unrelated transplantation [22]. However, private cord blood banks limit the access to cord blood transplant only to the donor or his/her relatives. As a consequence, commercial cord blood banks decrease the number of cord blood units suitable for allogenic unrelated transplantations with serious impacts on racial and ethnic minorities, which are usually underrepresented on donor registries internationally [12-14].

In light of these implications, this chapter aims to stimulate an ethical reflection on public and private cord blood banking, by focusing on the ethical duty and responsibility to give adequate, true and comprehensive information to expectant parents in order to facilitate an aware decision on newborn cord blood banking.

Public vs Private Cord Blood Banks: Numbers and Data

Public Cord Blood Banks

Since the first umbilical cord blood transplant (UCBT), performed in 1988 for the treatment of a child affected by Franconi Anemia, more than 20,000 allogenic cord blood transplantations have been reported worldwide and more than 600,000 cord blood units have been stored in public cord blood banks [1].

Cord blood transplants are now accepted as a standard option for the treatment of a variety of hematopoietic, immunologic and metabolic disorders [10].

As specified by Eliane Gluckman, the main practical advantages of using cord blood as an alternative source of stem cells are the a) relative ease of procurement, b) the absence of risks for mothers and baby donors, c) the reduced likelihood of transmitting infections and d) the ability to store fully tested and HLA typed transplants in a frozen state, available for immediate use [1].

Thanks to the biological characteristics of cord blood and the use of better banking techniques, there is currently an overall increase in annual CBT [23-24] and, in some transplant centers, cord blood is equally indicated or even given priority over other sources of unrelated hematopoietic progenitor cells [25-27].

Public not-for-profit cord blood banks have significantly contributed to this improvement. Today there are more than 100 active cord blood banks worldwide, mainly based in Australia, Belgium, Brazil, France, Israel, Italy, Spain, United Kingdom, and the USA [11]. Moreover, a number of international networks have been created, including, among others, Netcord (http://www.netcord.org), Asia Cord (http://asiacord.org), and Bone Marrow Donors Worldwide (http://www.bmdw.org).

Public cord blood banks provide the collection, storage and supply of safe and high quality cord blood units for allogenic (related and unrelated) transplantation, and promote the use of cord blood and research on cord blood biology [10].

All of these services are provided completely free of charge and they are open to all patients who need a cord blood transplant. In fact, because umbilical cord blood is less sensitive to donor-host tissue mismatch than other stem cell sources, a large number of patients can benefit from a smaller donor pool [12]. In particular, the greater histocompatibility of cord blood transplants relative to BMT extends cord blood transplant access to racial and ethnic minorities which remain, to date, underrepresented on donor registries worldwide [8].

Private Cord Blood Banks

At the same time as the creation of public cord blood banks, a number of private banks have been established in many parts of the world, most notably in the USA, Europe, Central and South America and more recently in Australia, New Zealand, the Middle East, India and other parts of Asia [12].

Over the last 15 years, about 900,000 cord blood units have been stored privately for personal use, and about 100 autologous transplants have been performed worldwide [13].

Commercial cord blood banks usually provide, for a variable fee, the collection and storage of the newborn cord blood for potential autologous transplantation or for related use [12], for example in the USA, it is between 1000 to 2500 dollars.

In some cases, such as in New Zealand and Australia, private cord blood banks restrict the use of collected cord blood to the individual child and prohibit the use of banked units by a sibling or a relative [28].

Basically, commercial cord blood banks promote the storage of the newborn cord blood for the treatment of several diseases including cancer, bone marrow failure syndromes and genetic disorders. They also emphasize the chance to store newborn cord blood as “biological insurance” [12] for possible future stem cell therapy.

In spite of the variety of disorders listed from commercial cord blood banks for sponsoring the storage of the newborn cord blood for private use, clinical evidence supporting autologous cord blood collection is presently lacking [12-13].

As reported by Sullivan [12], so far the majority of cord blood transplants are sourced from unrelated donors through public cord blood banks. Based on data provided from Eurocord and multi-disease specific reports, the long-term survival after cord blood transplantation in both children and adults is now comparable to bone marrow transplantation, supporting the wider use of cord blood banking and transplant [29-32].

Contrarily, there is currently little clinical data supporting the private storage of the newborn cord blood for autologous transplantation. Despite the number of privately banked cord blood units used, only three published single-case reports of autologous cord blood transplants provided from commercial cord blood banks have been published [33-35].

Moreover, a survey involving pediatric stem cell physicians performing autologous cord blood transplants reported that private cord blood banking was not recommended unless there were ill siblings and the parents were of North European descent [36].

In light of these positions, there is presently no published peer-reviewed evidence supporting the commercial banking of cord blood for autologous transplant. However, scientific data clearly supports public cord blood storage due to the likelihood of clinical need, concern over latent diseases in cord blood units and quality of stored cord blood [13].

Public vs. Private Cord Blood Banks: Ethical Considerations

Both public and private cord blood banks provide the collection and storage of newborn cord blood for stem cell transplantation. While apparently public and private cord blood banks seem to offer the same service, in actual fact they do not.

Public cord blood banks are usually publicly funded institutions providing, free of charge, the collection and the storage of the newborn cord blood for allogenic (related or unrelated) transplantation. Allogenic cord blood transplants are internationally supported with clinical evidence and they are increasing worldwide. Unrelated cord blood transplants nowadays account for over 20% of all stem cell transplants (50% in Japan), and since 2005 more cord blood transplants have been done in adults than in children [37].

Private cord blood banks are typically commercial companies providing, for a variable fee, the collection and storage of newborn cord blood for autologous and/or related transplantation.

In spite of the marketing of private cord blood banks, there is presently no clinical evidence supporting the storage of the newborn cord blood for autologous transplant [12-14, 36]. As noted by Sullivan, compared to the number of cord blood units banked privately, "it is surprising that no commercial provider has ever published peer reviewed data on the number of cord blood stored, the number of the units used and the outcome of any autologous transplants". [12]

The absence of adequate peer-reviewed data supporting the services sponsored from private cord blood banks is not simply a scientific problem but it raises several ethical concerns.

The first ethical issue concerning commercial cord blood banks, versus public cord blood banks, relates to the ethical validity of the informed consent given from expectant parents to commercial providers in order to store their newborn's cord blood in view of a future autologous transplantation [12]. The second issue concerns the principle of justice and relates to the need of an equal distribution of available resources – namely, stored cord blood units – among patients awaiting a cord blood transplant worldwide [14], including racial and ethnic minorities.

Private Cord Blood Banks: Informed Consent Bias

According to the ethical principles governing the medical practice and the research involving humans [20, 21], the informed consent of patients or research subjects is valid when given by individuals free of coercion, competent to consent to and properly informed.

Whereas public cord blood banks usually follow a standardized process for obtaining the parents informed consent, requiring detailed information on the storage of the newborn cord blood [38], private cord blood banks generally use different informed consent processes which are critical, ethically, for two main reasons: the first is about the accuracy of information given to future parents. The second relates to the completeness of the provided information.

With regard to the adequacy of information given from commercial providers to expecting parents, the European Recommendation Rec (2004) 8 of the Committee of Ministers to member states on autologous cord blood banks states that "Where autologous cord blood banks are being established, the promotional material or information provided to families must be accurate and fully informed consent to cord blood storage must be obtained" [19].

In a systematic review reported by Sullivan [12], concerning the analysis of the information of the English websites of 148 private cord blood banks "a pattern of confusing and potentially misleading information" [12] related to the benefits of autologous and relative cord blood banking emerged. Usually, commercial cord blood banks publish similar lists of diseases treatable through cord blood transplants, including cancer, genetic disorders, and bone marrow failure syndromes. Most private banks also list many conditions that might be treated in the future through advances in regenerative medicine.

The critical aspect of this information, in ethical terms, is the fact that they are not presently based on clinical evidence. As reported in the previous paragraph of this chapter, so far there is not adequate peer-reviewed data supporting the private storage of newborn cord blood for autologous transplant. On one hand, available reports on stored and used cord blood units for autologous transplantation are not enough to be considered as clinical evidence [12, 14]. On the other, among physicians performing autologous cord blood transplantation, it is not recommended to privately store newborn cord blood when there are no ill siblings and the parents are of North European descent.

Therefore, information provided by commercial cord blood banks to families is not completely accurate and consequently the consent given from parents to store the newborn cord blood for private use is not fully informed.

Moreover, information provided from private cord blood banks is often incomplete, rather than inaccurate. As previously mentioned, usually commercial cord blood banks provide similar lists of diseases treatable by umbilical cord blood transplants. Most of these disorders are treatable only with an allogenic (related or unrelated) cord blood transplant. However, many private banks do not explain clearly the difference between autologous and allogenic cord blood transplantation, leaving expectant parents to suppose that indications for allogenic transplantations also apply to autologous transplants [12].

Private Cord Blood Banks: Loss of Chances for Racial and Ethnic Minorities

Private storage of newborn cord blood for autologous transplantation also has detrimental effects on the likelihood of patients who need a CBT to find a suitable match. This particularly affects racial and ethnic minorities, usually underrepresented on the bone marrow registries worldwide [1, 12, 14].

As reported by Sullivan [12], although a unrelated matched donor can be found for up to 75% of patients of Western European origin, for many ethnic groups the reverse is true with no more than 20-30% being matched, leaving a number of patients with neither a related sibling donor nor an unrelated bone marrow donor [39-40].

Public cord blood banks, providing cord blood for allogenic transplantation, contribute to overcome this problem, allowing a great number of patients to benefit from a smaller donor pool.

On the contrary, private cord blood banks decrease the number of cord blood units available for allogenic transplantation with serious effects on patients of racial and ethnic minorities. Indeed, they are less likely to find matches for several reasons, including relative representation in donor registries and the increased genetic diversity with many low frequency HLA types found in patients of African origin [36].

Private cord blood banks come to strike the ethical principle of justice based on which mechanisms should be created to ensure that all potential participants in umbilical cord banking, including minorities, have equal access to cord blood transplants [14].

Conclusion

Public cord blood banks currently represent a precious source of cord blood units available for allogenic (related and unrelated) transplantation worldwide. Public cord blood banks offer safe and high quality services completely free of charge. They also give all patients needing a stem cell transplant the chance to find a suitable donor in volunteer registries, allowing racial and ethnic minorities to have equal access to cord blood transplants. Public cord blood banks reply to several ethical needs including solidarity, justice and respect of donor autonomy.

Private cord blood banks promote, for a variable fee, services that are not presently supported by clinical evidence. They often provide to expectant parents information lacking accuracy and completeness. They also limit the access to cord blood transplantation only to the donor or his/her relatives.

Based on existing data [12-14], private cord blood banks raise ethical concerns regarding the principle of autonomy and justice. On one hand, commercial cord blood banks usually do not provide truthful and complete information to expectant parents and consequently they do not facilitate an aware informed consent. On the other, private cord blood banks limit the likelihood of patients to find a suitable match with serious effects on racial and ethnic minorities which are still underrepresented on donor registries worldwide.

In light of this scenario, where multiple factors (for example, clinical data, ethical values, personal wishes) play a key role on the decision making process concerning the storage of newborn cord blood for public or private use, official declarations on cord blood banking would contribute to clarify this process.

So far, many ethical and medical organizations as well as policy makers, including the European Union Group on the Ethics and Science in Technology [18], the European Committees of Ministers to Member States (19), the American Academy of Pediatrics [9], the American College of Obstetricians and Gynaecologists [15-16] and the World Marrow Donor Associations [17] criticize private cord blood banks due to the present lack of scientific evidence supporting the storage of cord blood for autologous use. They also disapprove of commercial cord blood banks because of the negative effects that private cord blood banking has on altruistic donation.

Moreover, recent studies [41] reporting promising outcomes associated with the use of non-hematopoietic stem cells for the treatment of several diseases including, among others, diabetes, neurological disorders and myocardial infarction seem to encourage the storage of the newborn cord blood for allogenic transplantation.

References

[1] Gluckman E. Milestones in umbilical cord blood transplantation. *Blood Reviews*, 2011, 25, 255-259.

[2] Brunstein CG. Umbilical cord blood transplantation for the treatment of hematologic malignancies. *Cancer control*, 2011, 18, 222-236.

[3] Smith AR, Wagner JE. Alternative hematopoietic stem cell sources for transplantation: place of umbilical cord blood. *Br J Haematol*, 2009, 147, 246-261.

[4] Hwang WY, Samuel M, Tan D et al. A meta-analysis of unrelated donor umbilical cord blood transplantation versus unrelated donor bone marrow transplantation in adult and pediatric patients. *Bio Blood Marrow Transplant*, 2007, 13, 444-453.

[5] 5 unrelated donor umbilical cord blood and bone marrow in children with acute leukaemia: a comparison study (see comment). *Lancet*, 2007, 369, 1947-1954.

[6] Ponce DM, Zheng J, Gonzales AM et al. Reduced late mortalities risk contributes to similar survival after double-unit cord blood transplantation compared with related and unrelated donor hematopoietic stem cell transplantation. *Bio Blood Marrow Transplant,* 2011, 17, 316-1326.

[7] Brunstein CG, Gutman JA, Weisdor DJ et al. Allogenic hematopoietic cell transplantation for hematologic malignancies: relative risks and benefits of double umbilical cord blood. *Blood*, 2010, 116, 4693-4699.

[8] Barker JN, Byam CE, Kernan NA et al. Availability of cord blood extends allogenic hematopoietic stem cell transplant access to racial and ethnic minorities. *Bio Blood Marrow Transplant,* 2010 16, 1541-1548.

[9] American Academy of Pediatrics: Work Group on Cord Blood Banking: Cord blood banking for potential future transplantation: Subject Review. *Pediatrics*, 1999, 104(1), 116-118.

[10] Garcia J. Allogenic unrelated cord blood banking worldwide: An update. *Transfusion and Apheresis Science*, 2010, 42, 257-263.

[11] European Blood and Marrow Transplant Group. Activity survey. http://www.ebmt.org/4Registry

[12] Sullivan MJ. Banking on cord blood stem cells. *Nature Reviews Cancer*, 2008, 8, 554-563.

[13] Ballen K. Challenges in umbilical cord blood stem cell banking for stem cell reviews and reports. *Stem Cell Rev and Rep*, 2010, 6, 8-14.

[14] Broder SM Ponsaran RS Goldenberg AJ. US public cord blood banking: recruitment, donation, and the timing of consent. *Transfusion*, 2012, doi: 10.1111/j.1537-2995.2012.03785.x.

[15] American College of Obstetricians and Gynaecologists. Committee on Obstetric Practice; Committee on Genetics; ACOG committee opinion No 399: umbilical cord blood banking. *Obstet Gynecol*, 2008, 111, 475-477.

[16] American College of Obstetricians and Gynaecologists. Routine storage of umbilical cord blood for potential future transplantation. *Int J Gynaecol Obstet*, 1997, 57 257-259.

[17] American Medical Association. Opinion 2.165 - Umbilical Cord Blood Banking. 2008. *http://www.ama-assn.org/ama/pub/physician-resources/medical-ethics/code-medical-ethics/opinion2165.page*

[18] European Group on Ethics in Science and New Technologies (EGE) Ethical aspects of umbilical cord blood banking European Commission http://ec.europa.eu/european group_ethics/publications/docs/publop19_en.pdf(2004)

[19] Council of Europe. Recommendation Rec (2004) 8 of the Committee of Ministers to member states on autologous cord blood banks. 2004, https://wcd.coe.int/ViewDoc.jsp?id=744641&Lang=en

[20] Beauchamp TL, Childress JF. Principles of biomedical ethics. 2001, Oxford University Press.

[21] Engelhardt HT. The foundation of bioethics. 1986, 1996. Oxford University Press.

[22] Anasetti C, Aversa F, Brunstein CG. Back to the future: mismatched unrelated donor, haploidentical related donor, or unrelated umbilical cord blood transplantation? *American Society for Blood and Marrow Transplantation*, 2012 doi:10.1016/j.bbmt.2011.11.004

[23] Gluckman E, Rocha V. Donor selection for unrelated cord blood transplants. *Curr Opin Immunol,* 2006, 18, 565-570.

[24] Organizazion Nacional ded transplantes. Memoria de transplante de progenitors hemopoyeticos 2005 http: //www.ont.es/Estadistica in Garcia J, cit. (see reference 10).

[25] Sanz GF. Unrelated donor umbilical cord blood transplantation in adults with hematologic malignancies. *Pathol Biol*, 2005, 53, 165-166.

[26] Takahashi S, Iseki T, OOi J et al. Single-institute comparative analysis of unrelated bone marrow transplantation and cord blood transplantation for adult patients with hematologic malignancies. *Blood*, 2004, 104, 3813-3820.

[27] Gluckman E. Ten years of cord blood transplantations: from bench to bedside. *Br J Haematol,* 2009, 147, 192-199.

[28] Sullivan M, Browett P, Patton N. Private umbilical cord blood banking: a biological insurance of dubious future benefit. *NZ Med J,* 2005, 118U1, 260.

[29] Benito AI, Diaz MA, Gonzales VM et al. Hematopoietic stem cell transplantation using umbilical cord blood progenitors: review of current clinical results. *Bone Marrow Transplant*, 2004 35 675-690.

[30] Eapen M, Rubinstein P, Zhang MJ. Outcomes of transplantation of unrelated donor umbilical cord blood and bone marrow in children with acute leukaemia: a comparison study. *Lancet*, 2007, 369, 1947-1954.

[31] Rocha V, Cornish J, Sievers EL et al. Comparison of outcomes of unrelated bone marrow and umbilical cord blood transplants in children with acute leukaemia. *Blood*, 2001, 97, 2962-2971.

[32] Rocha V, Labopin M, Sanz G et al. Transplants of umbilical cord blood or bone marrow from unrelated donors in adults with acute leukaemia. *N Eng J Med*, 2004, 351, 2276-2285.

[33] Ferreira E, Pasternak J, Bacal N et al. Autologous cord blood transplantation. *Bone Marrow Transplant,* 1999, 24, 1041.

[34] Friedrich MJ. Growing role for umbilical cord blood. *JAMA*, 2004, 292, 2453-2454.

[35] Hayani A, Lampeter E, Viswanatha D et al. First report of autologous cord blood transplantation in the treatment of a child with leukaemia. *Pediatrics*, 2007, 119, e296-3007.

[36] Thornely I, Eapen M, Sung L et al. Private cord blood banking: experiences and views of pediatric hematopoietic cell transplantation physicians. *Pediatrics*, 2009, 123, 1011-1017.

[37] Shoemans H, Theunissen K, Maertens J et al. Adult umbilical cord blood transplantation: a comprehensive review. *Bone Marrow Transplant*, 2006, 38, 83-93.

[38] Petrini C. Umbilical cord blood collection, storage and use: ethical issues. Blood Transfusions, 2010, 139-148.

[39] Rubinstein P. Why cord blood? *Human Immunol*, 2006, 67, 398-404.

[40] van Rood JJ, Oudshoorn M. Eleven million donors in Bone Marrow Donors Worldwide! Time for reassessment? *Bone Marrow Transplant*, 2008, 41, 1-9.

[41] Kogler G, Sensken S Airey JA et al. A new human somatic stem cell from placental cord blood with intrinsic pluripotent differentiation potential. *J Exp Med*, 2004, 200, 123-135.

In: Cord Blood
Editor: Lisandra Vanostrand
ISBN: 978-1-62618-072-7

Chapter 5

CCR5 Deficient Cord Blood as a Means of Treatment of HIV-1 Infection

Gero Hütter*
Institute of Transfusion Medicine and Immunology,
Medical Faculty Mannheim, Heidelberg University,
German Red Cross Blood Service Baden-Württemberg, Hessen, Germany

Abstract

Infection with the human immunodeficiency virus type 1 (HIV-1) causes a continuous decrease of T-cells ending in the acquired immune deficiency syndrome (AIDS). HIV-1 requires the presence of a CD4 receptor and a chemokine receptor, namely CCR5. The most encouraging method of interrupting the interaction of the viral surface glycoprotein gp120 with this coreceptor involves the replacement of wild-type CCR5 with a truncated form of the receptor encoded by a 32 base-pair deletion (CCR5-delta32) in the CCR5 gene. Recently, the successful stem cell transplantation (SCT) of an HIV-1-infected patient suffering from acute myeloid leukemia, applying homozygous CCR5-delta32 donor cells has been reported. These hematopoietic progenitor cells engrafted, proliferated, and differentiated to produce mature myeloid and lymphoid

* E-mail: Gero.huetter@medma.uni-heidelberg.de.

cells that were highly resistant to HIV-1 infection. Currently, over 5 years after the transplantation and in the absence of any antiretroviral treatment, no plasma viral load or proviral DNA are detectable in peripheral blood cells and certain tissue samples in this patient. However, current attempts to repeat this approach failed due to the availability of matching CCR5 negative stem cell donors. To increase the probability in finding a matching donor Stemcyte and other facilities, built up databases with pretested umbilical cord blood units (UCB), genotyped for the CCR5-delta32 deletion. An international collaboration of HIV researches and transplant centers initiated in 2012 an initiative to carry on the idea of the use of UCB from CCR5-delta32 homozygous donors in patients with HIV requiring SCT.

Introduction

HIV-1 belongs to a subset of retroviruses called lentiviruses and is causative for AIDS. Infection with HIV-1 is characterized by the development of a global immune activation and a complex array of HIV-specific immune responses, resulting in a decrease in both, memory and naïve CD4+ T cells [1]. Due to the reduced number of CD4+ cells, patients are threatened by opportunistic infections and malignancies. Especially the rate of malignancies in patients with untreated HIV-infection is remarkable increased and became especially for B-non-Hodgkin´s lymphomas dramatically high [2, 3]. Even in the era of highly active antiretroviral therapy (HAART) the incidence of cancer is elevated in comparison to the HIV-negative population. Furthermore, some entities show clinically an unfavorable outcome in HIV+ patients, suggestions that there will be a rising demand for curative treatment options like high dose chemotherapy with allogeneic SCT in the future [4]. The exact number of HIV-patients who require allogeneic HSCT is not known but based on own experiences and epidemiological data we expect more than 30 transplants each year worldwide. In up to 20% related donors are available but in all other cases a search for an unrelated donor has to be performed.

The Principal Idea of HIV Treatment by Stem Cell Transplantation

The predominant target-cells of HIV-1 are CD4+ T-cells and macrophages, respectively. However, HIV is able to infect several bone marrow derived cells. The progressive clinical course of HIV-infection is characterized by an unrelenting devastation of CD4+ T-cells leading to AIDS and finally to death of the patient. Therefore, HIV-infection shares some characteristics with certain hematological diseases where SCT is often the only curative option in these patients.

Furthermore, HIV-1 can persist in a latent form in resting memory CD4+ cells carrying an integrated copy of the HIV genome. Because of these stable reservoir cells, eradication by antiretroviral therapy is unlikely and for eradication, alternative treatment options are required [5].

The first experimental attempt to affect the HIV-infection by SCT was made in the early 80´s by Hassett and coworkers by transfusion of large amounts of allogeneic T cells and CD34+ stem cells. Clinically the patients did not substantially improve from this procedure and the immunological condition remained only for a short time stable and than worsened [6]. Because of the impaired immune system in HIV+ individuals there was a great anxiety in the past that allogeneic SCT -in case of HIV- would be an unforeseeable risk in these patients.

Now, retrospective analysis of reported cases indicate that the outcome of allografted HIV positive patients is probably only negligible poorer, in comparison to HIV negative patients [7].

However, SCT alone is not sufficient to improve the course of HIV-1 infection because the of the re-infection of the new arising immune system due to the latently infected host cells which commonly survive the transplantation procedure.

A promising solution for this problem has been given after zidovudine received approval for HIV treatment in 1987. There was some hope that a suppression of viral replication by antiretroviral medication during the set up of allogeneic SCT might protect the arising new immune system from re-infection. And indeed, this theory followed a first encouraging case reported from Holland and coworkers in 1989.

A 41-year old man with refractory lymphoma underwent allogeneic SCT with concomitant zidovudine medication where HIV-RNA PCR was positive until day +32, and HIV culture experiments remained negative from day +25. Unfortunately, the patient died on day +47 after allogeneic SCT due to a relapse of his lymphoma [8].

However, it was not possible to repeat this observation in other SCT patients ongoing HAART.

The Role of the Transplantation Procedure

The transplantation procedure prior and after stem cell administration, consists in a combination of chemotherapy, irradiation, and a panel of immunosuppressive medications like anti-thymocyteglobuline (ATG) and cyclosporine A (CsA). Since 1983 over 60 cases of allogeneic stem cell transplantation in patients with HIV have been reported [9]. In all cases a combination of conditioning regimen and immuno-suppression has been performed. However, in only two patients an effect on HIV was suggested, but both passed away shortly after transplantation and no follow-up data were available.

ATG contains functional antibodies against T cell markers including CD4, CCR5 and CXCR4 resulting in a depletion of HIV-1 target cells. Recently, it has been demonstrated that ATG causes a long-lasting reduction of CD4+ T cells in HIV+ patients receiving HAART after renal transplant [10]. However, this CD4+ depletion had no effect on the course of infection or replication of HIV-1. Nevertheless, it can be suggested that ATG is capable in reducing the viral reservoir by depletion of infected CD4+ T cells and non-infected target cells during the period of application.

CsA was also tested during primary HIV-infection where it was not detrimental to virus-specific CD8+ or CD4+ T cell responses. A rapid shutdown of T cell activation in the early phases of primary HIV-1 infection may have long-term beneficial effects and establish a more favourable immunologic set-point. However, the activity of CsA and other immune-based therapeutic interventions during HIV infection are not sufficient to reduce the viral reservoir [11].

Another commonly used agent for immuno-suppression is mycophenolic mofetil (MMF) which acts as a selective and reversible inhibitor of de novo synthesis of deoxyguanosine triphosphate (dGTP). MFF's effects are selective for lymphocytes, and it suppresses HIV replication by depletion of substrates for reverse transcription. In addition, the MMF induced depletion of activated $CD4^+$ T cells reduces the number of target cells for HIV-1 replication through guanine depletion. It has been hypothesized that MMF could improve suppression of viral replication in the setting of low-level viremia. In a study with six HIV+ patients ongoing HAART and additionally MMF, authors found a correlation to viremia decline. Associated with sub optimal treatment adherence, clinical responses were not durable and the virostatic effect disappeared after discontinuation of MMF [12].

Taken together, allogeneic stem cell transplantation itself or concomitant medication due to the transplantation procedure have no sustained effect on viral replication nor have been found the be sufficient to decrease the HIV reservoir. In all cases HAART was interrupted a rapid rebound of HIV was observed.

A Case of "Natural" Gene Therapy

CCR5 and CXCR4 have been identified as two major coreceptors for entry of HIV-1 into host cells [13]. CCR5-tropic (R5) virus variants are usually responsible for the initial infection, while CXCR4 (X4) or dual tropic variants are often associated with late stages of the chronic infection [14]. Furthermore, the inflammatory response and recruitment of auxiliary CCR5 expressing cells in mucosal tissues is an important mechanism of transmission and a possible explanation of the preference of R5 variants during first infection [15].

A 32-basepair deletion in the CCR5 allele (CCR5-delta32) leads to a truncated gene product and provides resistance against HIV-1 transmission in individuals homozygous for this mutation [16]. Individuals homozygous for the CCR5-delta32 deletion can only be infected by non-CCR5-using strains like X4 variants that utilize CXCR4 as a coreceptor which is reported in some rare cases. Taken together, the CCR5-delta32 deletion provides a nearly complete protection against HIV transmission.

In February 2007, a medical team of the Charité Berlin performed an SCT in an HIV infected patient with acute myeloid leukaemia (AML) using progenitor cells from a donor especially selected to be homozygous for the CCR5-delta32 deletion. Allogeneic transplantation led to a change in the patients´ CCR5 allele genotype and finally, HIV remained undetectable for more than 5 years after discontinuing antiretroviral therapy, as determined by viral RNA and proviral DNA PCR assays of peripheral blood, bone marrow, and several tissue biopsies including gut and brain. Interestingly, although antiretroviral medication was stopped the day of SCT and proviral DNA was detectable in peripheral blood cells for 60 days after transplantation, no viral rebound was observed. More over, there was a discrepancy of residual CCR5 expression in different anatomical compartments. Whereas the proportion of CD4+/CCR5+ T cells in the peripheral blood declined from month to month,

CCR5 expression macrophages in the gut were still detectable half a year after transplantation. Finally, during a follow up period of currently five years, even these residual CCR5 expressing macrophages as a potential reservoir for latently infected cells became undetectable in certain tissues as determined by immunofluorescence histology [17, 18].

This unique case has encouraged further treatment regimens with the target of an HIV cure. In November 2010, the International AIDS Society (IAS) Governing Council prioritized an HIV cure as one of the organization's four key policy areas that align with its 2010 – 2014 strategic plan. Furthermore, approaches to knock-down CCR5 by gene techniques have been supported by the publicity of this –so called- "Berlin patient". Sangamo, with its zinc-finger nuclease (ZFN) based approach, has already published several small phase 1 trials using ZFN-mediated gene disruption technology to knock-down the CCR5 gene in cells of a patient's immune system to make these cells permanently resistant to HIV infection. However, the results of the first trials are preliminary and more experiences have to be collected for further conclusions concerning efficacy and safety of this approach [19, 20].

Attempts to Repeat the "Berlin Patient" Case

Taken together, over 16.000.000 people are already registered world wide as stem cell donors. Based on a 10/10 allele HLA-match, the probability in finding a matching donor is over 80%. Furthermore, commonly more than 1 donor and sometimes more than 100 donors are available for each patient. According to the frequency of around 1% homozygous CCR5-delta32 people there is a small but notable chance to find both, an HLA-identical and CCR5-depleted donor.

The major limitation is, that donors are generally not been tested concerning CCR5 and that testing from stored samples is not allowed. So, donors have to be informed, blood sample have to be obtained and tested. Furthermore, the large number of donors is distributed on hundreds of registries in different countries. In case of an HIV+ patient requiring unrelated SCT, there is simply not enough time to extend the donor search to the CCR5 typing [21].

One solution would be to test stem cell donors routinely, which is already a standard procedure in our Red Cross Stem Cell Registry (supported by a grant from the Bill & Melinda Gates Foundation). From March 2009 until now, our research group received 14 requests of HIV+ patients concerning CCR5-delta32 donors (update from [22]). Only in one search a homozygous donor was found, unfortunately the patient died due his malignancies before transplantation. In all other cases there were no matching donors available although in some case more than 100 were registered, or screening was interrupted because patient was in need of treatment due to disease progression. This limitation of time is one of the major obstacles in finding CCR5-delta32 homozygotes in unrelated donors.

Taken together, stem cell registries contain a large number of appropriate CCR5-depleted donors (160.000 compared to "only" 300 in all cord blood banks), however there is a limitation concerning rapid access to those units.

Use of Cord Blood for Allogeneic SCT

For patients with malignancies requiring SCT lacking a matched related or unrelated donor, UCB administration is viable option. For allogeneic SCT from adult donors a 10/10 allelic HLA match is commonly required. Using UCB units, there not such stringent HLA matching required. Acceptable HLA-matched units include those that are matched at 4 of 6, 5 of 6, or 6 of 6 alleles at 3 loci using low resolution testing at the A and B loci and high resolution testing at the DRB1 locus, disallowing 2 mismatches at the same locus for 4 of 6 matching. There are several trials that UCB transplantation is not inferior to hoploidentical transplantation. In comparison the HLA matched related or unrelated SCT, UCB transplantation provides similar response and progression-free survival rates with a reduced chronic graft-versus-host disease frequency. Only the treatment related mortality especially in terms of infectious complications is somehow higher compared to adult SCT [23-25].

CCR5 Negative Cord Blood for HIV+ Patients

In 2001 R. Chow (founder of StemCyte Inc.) and L. Petz built up a database with more than 25.000 cord blood units, genotyped for the CCR5-delta32 deletion. Chow´s group suggested that CCR5 negative cord blood units could be a potential source for the future HIV+ patients requiring allogeneic transplantation [26]. A similar approach was prepared by the M.D. Anderson CB Bank (Houston, Texas, USA), who have collected and CCR5-genotyped more than 10 000 cord blood units since 2005 [27].

Taken together over 300 of CCR5 negative UCB units are already pretested and registered. This would be sufficient to provide a 4/6 HLA matched unit with a 73.6% probability to Caucasian paediatric patients and 27.9% or Caucasian adults in the case that a minimal cell dose of $\geq 2.5 \times 10^7$ total nucleated cell count (TNC) /kg is accepted.

However, since the Stemcyte started the CCR5 testing in 2001 no CCR5-depleted UCB unit was administered until 2011. The reason for that is probably the good access to perfect matched stem cells from adult donors. Some countries, like Germany, do not use UCB in mentionable amounts. Some transplant centers are anxious that a delayed engraftment of UCB and the consecutive higher risk of opportunistic infections during aplasia would narrow the success of the transplant procedure.

To overcome these limitations, strategies to increase to probability of administration of UCB are required. One option could be the "dual transplant" method consisting in the co-infusion of only one UCB unit and a relatively low number of highly T-depleted mobilized CD34+ cells from an adult third party donor, after myeloablative conditioning regimen [28]. This approach has several advantages:

1. high accessibility of a haplo-donor.
2. increasing the probability of finding matching UCB due to the reduction of the required CD34+ cell dose. Lowering the required cell dose from 2.5 to 1.0×10^7 TNC/kg will increase the probability from 27.9% to 82.1% in adults.
3. reduced time of aplasia due to the haplo proportion of the transplant.
4. finally, after engraftment of the UCB unit will take over the myeloid function while the haplo part disappears after a couple of time resulting in a 100% chimerism of CCR5 depleted and HIV resistant peripheral blood cells.

This approach has been already performed in some selected patients (publication of first results is in progress) [29, 30]. Unfortunately, one of these patients died already 2½ months after transplantation procedure due to relapse of the malignancy (personal communication with Prof. Diez-Martin, Madrid, Spain). However, based on the principal concept, amfAR (The Foundation of AIDS Research) initiated an international think-thank in September 2012 in

Amsterdam to discuss the current state of allogeneic transplantation of CCR5-depleted stem cells in HIV+ patients. Due to the difficulties to find a second candidate for SCT from an adult unrelated donor, the meeting suggested to initiate a program to promote the idea of combined haplo/CCR5-negative UCB based on the experiences of the University of Utrecht, Netherlands (meeting report in progress) [31].

Limitations of the CCR5-delta32 Approach

During transmission of HIV CCR5 is the preferred coreceptor for cell entry. During time of infection, HIV is able to change its tropism to other chemokine coreceptors especially CXCR4. It is very obvious that homozgyosity toward CCR5-delta32 deletion provides a high degree of resistance against HIV transmission but the role of CCR5 during maintaining HIV infection is still unclear. The "Berlin patient" harbored an CXCR4 tropic variant before transplantation which did not emerge after CCR5 was withdrawn, a phenomenon which could not be really explained, yet [32]. As long as the circumstances of the success of the "Berlin patient" are not defined, it is not clear whether repeating this attempt will always lead to the same result.

Secondly, there is a broad discussion about sterilizing cure in the "Berlin patient". However, current investigations and several attempts with different techniques from tissues, cerebral fluid, and blood have failed to answer this question. According to the work of the Yukl/Deeks group, the current results of these testing are contradicting and incoherent. After all, both, confirming and disconfirming of a sterilizing cure of the "Berlin patient" has failed. However, the patient is well, now nearly 6 years off antiretroviral medication, without HIV related symptoms, without viral replication showing a perfect clinical remission of the infection which could be also the major aim in using the CCR5-based UCB approach rather than struggling for a sterilizing cure [33].

Conclusion and Outlook

Techniques, availability, and acceptance of the use of UCB as source for allogeneic SCT are growing. Patients with HIV have an increased risk for several malignancies and therefore are also candidates for allogeneic treatment regimes. Based on prior experiences in using CCR5 depleted stem cells during transplantation, there is a good chance to find more appropriate patients with HIV, who benefit from an administration of CCR5-negative UCB units. Current first single center experiences are not published so far. An international initiative by amfAR will probably give us the chance to include more patients into the CCR5-negative UCB approach and to collect more information which is also useful in autologous settings like gene therapy and ZFN techniques.

References

[1] Fauci A. S., Pantaleo G., Stanley S., Weissman D. Immunopathogenic mechanisms of HIV infection. *Ann Intern Med* 1996 Apr 1;124(7):654-63.

[2] Besson C., Goubar A., Gabarre J., Rozenbaum W., Pialoux G., Chatelet F. P. et al. Changes in AIDS-related lymphoma since the era of highly active antiretroviral therapy. *Blood* 2001 Oct 15;98(8):2339-44.

[3] Goedert J. J. The epidemiology of acquired immunodeficiency syndrome malignancies. *Semin Oncol* 2000 Aug;27(4):390-401.

[4] Haioun C., Lepage E., Gisselbrecht C., Bastion Y., Coiffier B., Brice P., et al. Benefit of autologous bone marrow transplantation over sequential chemotherapy in poor-risk aggressive non-Hodgkin's lymphoma: Updated results of the prospective study LNH87-2. Groupe d'Etude des Lymphomes de l'Adulte. *J Clin Oncol* 1997 Mar;15(3):1131-7.

[5] Siliciano J. D., Siliciano R. F. A long-term latent reservoir for HIV-1: discovery and clinical implications. *J Antimicrob Chemother* 2004 Jul;54(1):6-9.

[6] Hassett J. M., Zaroulis C. G., Greenberg M. L., Siegal F. P. Bone marrow transplantation in AIDS. *N Engl J Med* 1983 Sep 15; 309 (11): 665.

[7] Hütter G., Zaia J. A. Allogeneic haematopoietic stem cell transplanta-tion in patients with human immunodeficiency virus: the experiences of more than 25 years. *Clin Exp Immunol* Mar;163(3):284-95.

[8] Holland H. K., Saral R., Rossi J. J., Donnenberg A. D., Burns W. H., Beschorner W. E. et al. Allogeneic bone marrow transplantation, zidovudine, and human immunodeficiency virus type 1 (HIV-1) infection. Studies in a patient with non-Hodgkin lymphoma. *Ann Intern Med* 1989 Dec 15;111(12):973-81.

[9] Hütter G., Zaia J. A. Allogeneic haematopoietic stem cell transplantation in patients with human immunodeficiency virus: the experiences of more than 25 years. *Clin Exp Immunol* 2011 Mar; 163 (3):284-95.

[10] Carter J. T., Melcher M. L., Carlson L. L., Roland M. E., Stock P. G. Thymoglobulin-associated Cd4+ T-cell depletion and infection risk in HIV-infected renal transplant recipients. *Am J Transplant* 2006 Apr; 6 (4):753-60.

[11] Rizzardi G. P., Harari A., Capiluppi B., Tambussi G., Ellefsen K., Ciuffreda D. et al. Treatment of primary HIV-1 infection with cyclosporin A coupled with highly active antiretroviral therapy. *J Clin Invest* 2002 Mar;109(5):681-8.

[12] Kaur R., Bedimo R., Kvanli M. B., Turner D., Shaw L., Margolis D. A placebo-controlled pilot study of intensification of antiretroviral therapy with mycophenolate mofetil. *AIDS Res Ther* 2006;3:16.

[13] Pierson T. C., Doms R. W. HIV-1 entry and its inhibition. *Curr Top Microbiol Immunol* 2003;281:1-27.

[14] Henry K. R., Weber J., Quinones-Mateu M. E., Arts E. J. The impact of viral and host elements on HIV fitness and disease progression. *Curr HIV/AIDS Rep* 2007 Feb;4(1):36-41.

[15] Li Q., Estes J. D., Schlievert P. M., Duan L., Brosnahan A. J., Southern P. J., et al. Glycerol monolaurate prevents mucosal SIV transmission. *Nature* 2009 Mar 4.

[16] Liu R., Paxton W. A., Choe S., Ceradini D., Martin S. R., Horuk R. et al. Homozygous defect in HIV-1 coreceptor accounts for resistance of some multiply-exposed individuals to HIV-1 infection. *Cell* 1996 Aug 9;86(3):367-77.

[17] Hütter G., Nowak D., Mossner M., Ganepola S., Mussig A., Allers K. et al. Long-term control of HIV by CCR5 Delta32/Delta32 stem-cell transplantation. *N Engl J Med* 2009 Feb 12;360(7):692-8.

[18] Allers K., Hütter G., Hofmann J., Loddenkemper C., Rieger K., Thiel E. et al. Evidence for the cure of HIV infection by CCR5Delta32/Delta32 stem cell transplantation. *Blood* 2011 Mar 10;117(10):2791-9.

[19] Perez E. E., Wang J., Miller J. C., Jouvenot Y., Kim K. A., Liu O. et al. Establishment of HIV-1 resistance in CD4+ T cells by genome editing using zinc-finger nucleases. *Nat Biotechnol* 2008 Jul;26(7):808-16.

[20] June C., Tebas P., Stein D., Mitsuyasu R., Lalezari J., Wang S. et al., editors. Induction of Acquired CCR5 Deficiency with Zinc Finger Nuclease-modified Autologous CD4 T Cells (SB-728-T) Correlates with Increases in CD4 Count and Effects on Viral Load in HIV-infected

Subjects. *19th Conference of Retroviruses and Opportunistic Infections*; 2012; Seattle, USA.

[21] Hütter G., Schneider T., Thiel E. Transplantation of selected or transgenic blood stem cells - a future treatment for HIV/AIDS? *J Int AIDS Soc* 2009;12:10.

[22] Hütter G., Thiel E. Allogeneic transplantation of CCR5-deficient progenitor cells in a patient with HIV infection: an update after 3 years and the search for patient no. 2. *AIDS* 2011 Jan 14;25(2):273-4.

[23] Ponce D. M., Zheng J., Gonzales A. M., Lubin M., Heller G., Castro-Malaspina H. et al. Reduced late mortality risk contributes to similar survival after double-unit cord blood transplantation compared with related and unrelated donor hematopoietic stem cell transplantation. *Biol Blood Marrow Transplant* 2011 Sep;17(9):1316-26.

[24] Sauter C., Abboud M., Jia X., Heller G., Gonzales A. M., Lubin M. et al. Serious infection risk and immune recovery after double-unit cord blood transplantation without antithymocyte globulin. *Biol Blood Marrow Transplant* 2011 Oct;17(10):1460-71.

[25] Smith A. R., Wagner J. E. Alternative haematopoietic stem cell sources for transplantation: place of umbilical cord blood. *Br J Haematol* 2009 Oct;147(2):246-61.

[26] Lawrence P., Istvan R., Yvonne B., Donna R., Joanne K., Elizabeth S. et al. Hematopoietic Cell Transplantation with Cord Blood for Cure of HIV Infections. *Biol Blood Marrow Transplant* 2012 Oct 19.

[27] Gonzalez G., Park S., Chen D., Armitage S., Shpall E., Behringer R. Identification and frequency of CCR5Delta32/Delta32 HIV-resistant cord blood units from Houston area hospitals. *HIV Med* 2012 Sep; 12 (8):481-6.

[28] Kwon M., Balsalobre P., Serrano D., Perez Corral A., Buno I., Anguita J. et al. Single Cord Blood Combined with HLA-Mismatched Third Party Donor Cells: Comparable Results to Matched Unrelated Donor Transplantation in High-Risk Patients with Hematologic Disorders. *Biol Blood Marrow Transplant* 2012 Sep 6.

[29] Kwon M., Serrano D., Balsalobre P., Anguita J., Buno I., P. M. et al., editors. A Single Cord Blood Transplantation Combined with a HLA Mismatched Third Party Donor for a Patuient with Burkitt Lymphoma and HIV Infection. *10th International Cord Blood Symposium*; 2012; San Francisco.

[30] Kuball J., editor. Towards the Next Generation of Transplantation: HIV Positive Patients. *10th International Cord Blood Symposium*; 2012; San Francisco.

[31] Johnston R., Collins C. Can we treat our way out of HIV? *AIDS Res Hum Retroviruses* 2012 Jan;26(1):1-4.

[32] Symons J., Deeks S. G., Hütter G., Wensing A. M. J., van Ham P. M., Vandekerckhove L. et al. Lack of X4-tropic HIV prevents viral rebound post CCR5-Δ32 Stem Cell Transplantation in the "Berlin Patient". *Plos One* 2013;[in progress].

[33] Yukl S., Deeks S. G., Boritz E., Busch M., Chun T., Douek D. et al. Challenges Inherent in Detecting HIV Persistence during Potentially Curative Interventions: a Study of the Berlin Patient. *PLOS Pathogens* 2013;[in progress].

In: Cord Blood
Editor: Lisandra Vanostrand

ISBN: 978-1-62618-072-7

Chapter 6

Therapeutic Use of Umbilical Cord Blood: Biology, Banking, and Ethical Issues

Sang Hun Lee, So Young Yoo and Sang Mo Kwon*

Laboratory for Vascular Medicine and Stem Cell Biology, Convergence Stem Cell Research Center, Department of Physiology, School of Medicine, Pusan National University, Yangsan, Korea

Abstract

Umbilical cord blood (UCB) is an alternative source to bone marrow or peripheral blood to obtain functional hematopoietic stem cells (HSCs) for transplantation to reconstitute the blood and immune system after myeloablative or radiation therapy for numerous malignant and nonmalignant conditions. Since the world's first UCB transplant was performed in 1988, over 10,000 UCB transplants have been conducted worldwide. The use of UCB is now expected to grow not only because more UCB units are available for traditional hematopoietic

* Corresponding author: Sang-Mo Kwon, PhD. Laboratory for Vascular Medicine and Stem Cell Biology, Research Institute of Convergence of Biomedical Science and Technology, Department of Physiology, School of Medicine, Pusan National University, Yangsan, Kore. Tel: 82-51-510-8070, Fax: 82-51-510-8076, E-mail: smkwon323@pusan.ac.kr, smkwon323 @hotmail.com.

transplantation but also because new stem cell therapies such as regenerative medicine have emerged into clinical applications.

This chapter summarizes UCB biology, storage methods for UCB banking, and current clinical applications, and it discusses ethical issues and risks.

Cord Blood Biology

Umbilical cord blood (UCB) may be used in traditional transplantation and may be applied in emerging clinical areas. UCB collected and stored at birth has advantages over bone marrow or peripheral blood, which generally is withdrawn much later in life, that are attributable to its immunological naivety. UCB-derived mononuclear cells (MNCs) are composed primarily of monocytes and lymphocytes. Lymphocytes of UCB are immunologically immature compared to those of bone marrow and peripheral blood. In addition, UCB-derived cells maintain higher ratios of naïve to memory $CD4^+$ and $CD8^+$ T cells, higher concentrations of natural killer cells (NK) cells, and lower concentrations of reactive natural killer T (NKT) cells than those of bone marrow and peripheral blood [1]. Cytokines are expressed at lower levels in UCB than in bone marrow and peripheral blood [2]. Anti-inflammatory cytokines are expressed at higher levels than pro-inflammatory cytokines in UCB. Therefore, the immunologically immature characteristics and anti-inflammatory properties of UCB both underlie the low frequency and reduced severity of graft-versus-host disease (GvHD) in allogeneic transplants, which may facilitate indirect cellular therapeutic benefits in regenerative medicine applications [1, 3].

The largest stem cells isolated from UCB are of the hematopoietic lineage that expresses the cell surface glycoprotein CD34, which constitutes approximately 1% of the MNCs in UCB [4]. The $CD34^+$ cell population is heterogeneous; it contains primitive cells and mature cells that differentiate along the hematopoietic lineage. UCB contains a higher percentage of primitive $CD34^+$ cells, such as pluripotent $CD34^+CD38^-$ and $CD34^+CD33^-$ cells, than bone marrow or peripheral blood [1]. These primitive $CD34^+$ cells are believed to enable long-term hematopoietic reconstitution in transplantation [1, 5]. UCB stem cells harbor greater pre-operative potential than bone marrow stem cells; UCB stem cell proliferation rates are reported to be as much as 8-fold greater than bone marrow stem cell proliferation rates. In addition, UCB reportedly consists of endothelial cell precursors, mesenchymal cell progenitors, and multipotent or pluripotent stem cells, which would be highly useful in regenerative medicine applications to treat damages associated with non-hematopoietic tissues [4].

Cord Blood Collection

UCB is generally collected following infant delivery either before or after placental delivery. UCB collected when the placenta is *in utero* has higher volumes and greater numbers of total nucleated cells (TNCs), $CD34^+$ cells, and colony-forming units (CFUs) [6] because the uterine contractions that occur when the placenta is *in utero* supposedly facilitate drawing of the blood, which improves the UCB collection volume. Collection methods include clamping and cutting the umbilical cord after delivery, disinfecting with alcohol or a betadine swab, and inserting the needle into the umbilical vein. Blood can be collected by active syringe withdrawal or a gravity bag. The collection volume and the number of TNCs and MNCs are reportedly higher in syringe-collected samples [7], although experienced collectors typically withdraw comparable volumes by either collection method and many obstetricians prefer the ease of the gravity bag. In addition to the collection method, obstetric factors such as gestation period (close to 40 weeks), higher birth weight, moderate maternal age (20–37 years), and fewer previous pregnancies have been associated with greater stem cell yield [8].

Cord Blood Banking

In the 1990s, the ability to collect and store UCB easily as a source of stem cells for transplantation without imparting risk to the child or mother led to the development of UCB banks [9]. Two types of UCB banks are available: public and private (or family). Public UCB banks operate similarly to blood banks, in which the donated UCB is stored for public use. Approximately 35 public banks exist worldwide and contain a combined total of 250,000 UCB units (estimate). The public UCB banking system intensively screens mothers who wish to donate for her medical history, high-risk behaviors, infectious disease, and, in some cases, inherited disease. Even after the mothers meet inclusion criteria, UCB from them also must meet the criteria of quality standards for cell number and volume prior to storage. Then, an estimated 65–

70% of units collected for public banks are discarded [10]. No fees are charged to donors for donating samples, but transplant hospitals are charged $15,000–$35,000 for sample retrieval by public banks [10]. Private banks store UCB for future use by the child from whose mother it was collected or by a relative (e.g., a sibling). Over 600,000 UCB units are stored in private banks worldwide [9]. Parents choose to bank the maternal UCB for their child for peace of mind, biological insurance, in the case of family history of a disease treatable by stem cells, adoption, mixed ethnicity, and as a genetically identical stem cell resource for future regenerative medicine applications.

UCB is collected by an obstetrician or midwife using collection kits provided by the bank. After it is collected, UCB is shipped to the bank for processing and storage. Private banks charge a fee of approximately $1500 for the initial collection and an annual storage fee of approximately $100 per year. Private banks are willing to store UCB for all parents who wish to store UCB with certain costs; there are no exclusion criteria or geographical barriers. Maternal blood samples are tested for infectious diseases including hepatitis B and C, human T-lymphotropic virus, cytomegalovirus, syphilis, and human immunodeficiency virus (HIV). Samples positive for infectious disease may be stored and kept on record according to the policies associated with each private bank. Generally, no costs are incurred to release the sample, but some private banks may charge processing or shipment fees. Some private banks have programs that enable UCB storage for directed donation at no cost if a relative has a disease that is treatable by stem cell transplantation.

Cord Blood Storage

Cryopreservation and thawing techniques have progressed considerably to maintain viable hematopoietic stem cells (HSCs) from bone marrow, peripheral blood, and UCB. Cord blood is cryopreserved in the liquid phase of liquid nitrogen by using techniques described by Rubinstein et al. [11]. Despite current technological advances, the period for which UCB remains viable after cryopreservation is uncertain. Broxmeyer et al. suggested that frozen cord blood can be stored and remains viable for 10–15 years, and functional stem cells needed for successful transplantation can be recovered from such frozen UCB with high efficiency [12, 13]. Most cord blood samples that are used clinically are the recovered after ≤6 years of cryopreservation. Thus, the engrafting capacity of cord blood stored for long periods must be confirmed with clinical results that demonstrate long-term, successful engraftment.

Clinical Applications

UCB has been successfully applied in HSC transplantation for malignant and non-malignant blood and bone marrow disorders. Diseases that are treatable with UCB stem cells include blood-related disorders, malignancies, and inherited metabolic and immune disorders as listed in Table 1. Unrelated UCB transplant outcomes reviewed by Brunstein and his colleagues showed that disease-free survival rates (1–3 years post-transplantation) for leukemia patients were 31–60% in children and 19–77% in adults [14]. For non-malignant conditions, the survival rates in children using unrelated UCB were 70–80% for immunodeficiency diseases [14] and 72% for metabolic storage diseases [15]. Fewer transplantations were conducted using related UCB transplants. Among them, most were applied to pediatric patients because of their access to related UCB samples. One early study reported significantly higher survival rates in recipients of related UCB transplants than in recipients of unrelated UCB transplants (63% versus 29%; $p < 0.001$) for the treatment of both malignancies and non-malignancies [16]. According to a Eurocord report for related UCB transplants over a 3-year-period, the survival rate was 71% for early-phase malignancies, 45% for intermediate-phase malignancies, 24% for advanced-phase malignancies, 82% for bone marrow failure disorders, 100% for hemoglobinopathies, and 70% for inborn errors of metabolism or primary immunodeficiencies [17]. The factors associated with UCB transplant outcomes include patient disease status, negative cytomegalovirus status, and the cell dose in the graft [18]. The majority of studies have found that increased cell dose, which is measured as TNCs, $CD34^{+}$, or CFU-granulocyte macrophages (CFU-GMs), imparts the greatest impact on engraftment and the subsequent transplant complications and survival.

Transplantation data acquired over the past 20 years reveal that UCB associates with significantly fewer GvHD complications than bone marrow and peripheral blood transplants. This likely contributes to the growing use of UCB because chronic GvHD is the leading cause of non-relapse–related mortality in transplantation [19]. Meta-analysis of UCB and bone marrow transplantation to treat malignant or non-malignant disease revealed similar survival rates but lower GvHD rates in both children and adults receiving UCB transplantation than those receiving bone marrow transplantation despite the high levels of human leukocyte antigen (HLA) disparity between UCB transplant donors and recipients [20]. In HLA-identical sibling donor transplantation, the use of UCB results in comparable survival rates to those resulting from bone marrow use, and significantly less acute and chronic GvHD occurs as an outcome of using UCB than bone marrow [21]. Related UCB transplantation appears to reduce GvHD risk (acute, by 3–20%; chronic, by 6–14%) compared to unrelated UCB transplants (acute, by 20–50%; chronic, by 5–30%) [14]. Interestingly, recipients of UCB transplant responded better to the treatment for chronic GvHD than recipients of bone marrow and peripheral blood transplants [22]. Peripheral blood allogeneic transplantations result in higher rates of GvHD than bone marrow transplantations [23].

Autologous HSC transplants carry far fewer complications than other transplants because of the decreased risk of immune complications, and they are often indicated in transplant situations. The immune complications by autologous HSC transplantation are indicated by acute myeloid leukemia, many forms of non-Hodgkin's lymphoma, myeloma, solid tumors, and autoimmune diseases (e.g., multiple sclerosis and Crohn's disease). Successful outcomes of autologous cord blood transplants have been reported for the treatment of neuroblastoma [24], aplastic anemia [25], and lymphoblastic leukemia [26]. The use of UCB in autologous transplantation is expected to grow as the private UCB banking industry grows and HSCs (without harvest complications) are readily provided by them for autologous transplant indications. The use of UCB provides several advantages over the use of bone marrow and peripheral blood in allogeneic and autologous transplantation (see Table 2). As discussed above, UCB transplants are less likely to result in GvHD, which enables greater immune tolerance of HLA disparities in allogeneic transplantation.

Siblings are twice as likely to be eligible for the UCB of one another as for bone marrow; UCB transplantation has been performed successfully with 1, 2, or even 3 HLA mismatches [26, 27], whereas bone marrow transplantation typically requires a perfect HLA match. UCB also maintains larger populations of CFU-GMs [28] and stem cells with relatively longer telomeres and increased proliferative potential than bone marrow. These characteristics appear to enhance the hematological and immunological reconstitution over the use of bone marrow.

A study by Frassoni and his colleagues observed higher numbers of committed and early progenitor cells in the bone marrow of children 1 year post-UCB transplantation than in bone marrow of children 1 year post-bone marrow transplantation [29].

In addition, the peripheral blood MNCs of UCB transplant recipients are reported to contain significantly longer telomeres than the peripheral blood MNCs of graft recipients, which suggests a replicative advantage of UCB stem cells [30]. The use of UCB is associated with a lower risk of viral contamination than bone marrow [31]. The ease and safety of UCB collection and its capacity for long-term storage provides the advantage of immediate availability for autologous and allogeneic clinical use. In contrast, in the case of bone marrow or peripheral blood transplants, the time required to search for a donor, locate the donor, establish the eligibility, and harvest the cells may result in disease relapse or progression and thus preclude transplant feasibility [17].

However, one disadvantage of UCB transplantation may be considered: the relatively low graft cell dose due to limitations of the collection volume. The cell dose affects the time necessary for hematological recovery. Several reports have shown that lower cell doses are associated with slower engraftment [18, 27, 32, 33].

For adult transplantation, cell dose is a major obstacle, compared to pediatric transplantation, because larger cell doses are needed for the hematological reconstitution of larger adult body masses. To overcome the cell dose issue in adults, 2 methods were proposed: the expansion of UCB stem cells and the use of multiple UCB units.

Despite the slow engraftment time, one study discovered that adult recipients of unrelated UCB transplants showed similar engraftment, treatment-related mortality, and disease-free survival rates as adults who received related bone marrow or peripheral blood [34].

Ethical Issues in Umbilical Cord Blood Banking

Many ethical questions remain unanswered with regard to the clinical and experimental use of UCB. These issues and needs include the development of ethical processes for donor recruitment and an informed consent procedure regarding cord blood banking and the process donating UCB to public banks, private banks, or for research purposes. Complex and controversial legal and ethical issues also merit to be mentioned: privacy, confidentiality, and ownership of cord blood units.

The questions of whether donor information must be associated with individual units of cord blood and whether donors should be informed of detected infections or genetic abnormalities are also controversial. The ethical aspects of commercial cord blood banking, particularly in terms of its clinical or experimental availability as a potentially valuable resource, are the subject of considerable debate.

Donor Recruitment

The parents of a child in gestation seek the best opportunities to ensure the child's health, and therefore, are vulnerable to promotional and advertising campaigns that inflate the potential benefits of UCB banking. Private banks market the collection and storage of UCB samples as biological insurance and argue for benefits that are not grounded in satisfactory scientific data. Commercial banks passionately describe UCB transplantation and emphasize its "vital importance" or "miraculous" benefits by utilizing various methods of communication such as the Internet, direct mail, and video. Public banks appeal to pregnant women to consider donating for altruistic reasons. However, for the recruitment process to be fair, donors must be informed accurately and impartially about the benefits and potential risks associated with UCB banking.

Messages creating a sense of guilt to parents who choose not to donate UCB should be denounced, and the decisional autonomy of parents should be preserved. Moreover, the use of coercive strategies to recruit UCB donors among ethnic minorities should be forbidden.

Conclusion

UCB is utilized increasingly in traditional HSC transplantations and is considered an ideal candidate for emerging stem cell therapies involved in regenerative medicine and gene therapy. UCB provides several advantages over other hematopoietic stem cell sources, such as easy harvest without risk to the donor, the provision of younger cells with longer telomeres and increased proliferative capacity, reduced likelihood of GvHD, the existence of a perfect genetic match that is stored for autologous use, and the ready availability for clinical use.

UCB can be collected at birth easily and stored in a public health bank for future use by the public or stored in a private bank for future use by the family or child from whom it was collected.

Although treatments are currently available only to children with stored UCB, the availability of autologous UCB units stored in private banks will allow more clients to participate in groundbreaking regenerative medicine. Given the medical significance of UCB, obstetricians should inform and discuss the options of private and public UCB banking with pregnant patients.

References

[1] Theilgaard-Mönch, K., Raaschou-Jensen, K., Palm, H., Schjødt, K., Heilmann, C., Vindeløv, L., Jacobsen, N., Dickmeiss, E. Flow cytometric assessment of lymphocyte subsets, lymphoid progenitors, and hematopoietic stem cells in allogeneic stem cell grafts. *Bone Marrow Transplant.* 2001 Dec.;28(11):1073-82

[2] Gluckman, E., Rocha, V., History of the clinical use of umbilical cord blood hematopoietic cells, *Cytotherapy*, 2005;7:219–27.

[3] Willing, A. E., Eve, D. J., Sanberg, P. R., Umbilical cord blood transfusions for prevention of progressive brain injury and induction of neural recovery: an immunological perspective, *Regen. Med.*, 2007;2: 457–64.

[4] Newcomb, J. D., Sanberg, P. R., Klasko, S. K., Willing, A. E., Umbilical cord blood research: current and future perspectives, *Cell Transplant*, 2007;16:151–8.

[5] Ueda, T., Yoshida, M., Yoshino, H., et al., Hematopoietic capability of CD34+ cord blood cells: a comparison with CD34+ adult bone marrow cells, *Int. J. Hematol.*, 2001;73:457–62.

[6] Solves, P., Mirabet, V., Planelles, D., et al., Influence of volume reduction and cryopreservation methodologies on quality of thawed umbilical cord blood units for transplantation, *Cryobiology*, 2008;56: 152–8.

[7] Skoric, D., Balint, B., Petakov, M., et al., Collection strategies and cryopreservation of umbilical cord blood, *Transfus. Med.*, 2007;17:107–13.

[8] McGuckin, C. P., Basford, C., Hanger, K., et al., Cord blood revelations: the importance of being a first born girl, big, on time and to a young mother!, *Early Hum. Dev.*, 2007;83:733–41.

[9] Goldstein, G., Toren, A., Nagler, A., Transplantation and other uses of human umbilical cord blood and stem cells, *Curr. Pharm. Des.*, 2007;13: 1363–73.

[10] Moise, K. J. Jr, Umbilical cord stem cells, *Obstet. Gynecol.*, 2005;106: 1393–1407

[11] Rubinstein, P., Dobrila, L., Rosenfield, R. E. Processing and cryopreservation of placental/ umbilical cord blood for unrelated bone marrow reconstitution. *Proc. Natl. Acad. Sci. US* 1995;92:10119–22.

[12] Broxmeyer, H. E., Cooper, S. High-efficiency recovery of immature hematopoietic progenitor cells with extensive proliferative capacity in human cord blood cryopreserved for 10 years. *Clin. Exp. Immunol.* 1997;107:45–53.

[13] Broxmeyer, H. E., Srour, E. F., Hangoc, G., Cooper, S., Anderson, S. A., Bodine, D. M. High-efficiency recovery of functional hematopoietic progenitor and stem cells from human cord blood cryopreserved for 15 years. *Proc. Natl. Acad. Sci. US* 2003;100:645–50.

[14] Brunstein, C. G., Setubal, D. C., Wagner, J. E., Expanding the role of umbilical cord blood transplantation, *Br. J. Haematol.*, 2007;137:20–35.

[15] Martin, P. L., Carter, S. L., Kernan, N. A., et al., Results of the cord blood transplantation study (COBLT): outcomes of unrelated donor umbilical cord blood transplantation in pediatric patients with lysosomal and peroxisomal storage diseases, *Biol. Blood Marrow Transplant*, 2006;12:184–94.

[16] Gluckman, E., Rocha, V., Boyer-Chammard, A., et al., Outcome of cordblood transplantation from related and unrelated donors. Eurocord Transplant Group and the European Blood and Marrow Transplantation Group, *N Engl. J. Med.*, 1997;337(6)373–81.

[17] Rocha, V., Locatelli, F., Searching for alternative hematopoietic stem cell donors for pediatric patients, *Bone Marrow Transplant*, 2008; 41: 207–14.

[18] Gluckman, E., Rocha, V., Arcese, W., et al., Factors associated with outcomes of unrelated cord blood transplant: guidelines for donor choice, *Exp. Hematol.*, 2004;32:397–407.

[19] Socie, G., Stone, J. V., Wingard, J. R., et al., Long-term survival and late deaths after allogeneic bone marrow transplantation. Late Effects

Working Committee of the International Bone Marrow Transplant Registry, *N Engl. J. Med.*, 1999;341:14–21.

[20] Hwang, W. Y., Samuel, M., Tan, D., et al., A meta-analysis of unrelated donor umbilical cord blood transplantation versus unrelated donor bone marrow transplantation in adult and pediatric patients, *Biol. Blood Marrow Transplant*, 2007;13:444–53.

[21] Rocha, V., Wagner, J. E. Jr, Sobocinski, K. A., et al., Graft-versus-host disease in children who have received a cord-blood or bonemarrow transplant from an HLA-identical sibling. Eurocord and International Bone Marrow Transplant Registry Working Committee on Alternative Donor and Stem Cell Sources, *N Engl. J. Med.*, 2000;342:1846–54.

[22] Arora, M., Nagaraj, S., Wagner, J. E., et al., Chronic graft-versus-host disease (cGVHD) following unrelated donor hematopoietic stem cell transplantation (HSCT): higher response rate in recipients of unrelated donor (URD) umbilical cord blood (UCB), *Biol. Blood Marrow Transplant,* 2007;13:1145–52.

[23] Cutler, C., Giri, S., Jeyapalan, S., et al., Acute and chronic graft-versushost disease after allogeneic peripheral-blood stem-cell and bone marrow transplantation: a meta-analysis, *J. Clin. Oncol.*, 2001;19:3685–91.

[24] Ferreira, E., Pasternak, J., Bacal, N., et al., Autologous cord blood transplantation, *Bone Marrow Transplant*, 1999;24:1041.

[25] Fruchtman, S. M., Hurlet, A., Dracker, R., et al., The successful treatment of severe aplastic anemia with autologous cord blood transplantation, *Biol. Blood Marrow Transplant*, 2004;10:741–2.

[26] Urban, C., Schwinger, W., Benesch, M., et al., Autologous cord blood transplantation in a child with acute lymphoblastic leukemia and central nervous system relapse, *Pediatrics*, 2007;119:1042–43, author reply 1043.

[27] Rubinstein, P., Carrier, C., Scaradavou, A., et al., Outcomes among 562 recipients of placental-blood transplants from unrelated donors, *N Engl. J. Med.,* 1998;339:1565–77.

[27] Wagner, J. E., Kernan, N. A., Steinbuch, M., et al., Allogeneic sibling umbilical-cord-blood transplantation in children with malignant and non-malignant disease, *Lancet*, 1995;346:214–19.

[28] Broxmeyer, H. E., Hangoc, G., Cooper, S., et al., Growth characteristics and expansion of human umbilical cord blood and estimation of its potential for transplantation in adults, *Proc. Natl. Acad. Sci. US,* 1992; 89:4109–13

[29] Frassoni, F., Podesta, M., Maccario, R., et al., Cord blood transplantation provides better reconstitution of hematopoietic reservoir compared with bone marrow transplantation, *Blood*, 2003;102:1138–41.
[30] Pipes, B. L., Tsang, T., Peng, S. X., et al., Telomere length changes after umbilical cord blood transplant, *Transfusion*, 2006;46:1038–43.
[31] Behzad-Behbahani, A., Pouransari, R., Tabei, S. Z., et al., Risk of viral transmission via bone marrow progenitor cells versus umbilical cord blood hematopoietic stem cells in bone marrow transplantation, *Transplant Proc*., 2005;37:3211–12.
[32] Iori, A. P., Cerretti, R., De Felice, L., et al., Pre-transplant prognostic factors for patients with high-risk leukemia undergoing an unrelated cord blood transplantation, *Bone Marrow Transplant*, 2004;33:1097–1105.
[33] Migliaccio, A. R., Adamson, J. W., Stevens, C. E., et al., Cell dose and speed of engraftment in placental/umbilical cord blood transplantation: graft progenitor cell content is a better predictor than nucleated cell quantity, *Blood*, 2000;96:2717–22.
[34] Takahashi, S., Ooi, J., Tomonari, A., et al., Comparative single-institute analysis of cord blood transplantation from unrelated donors with bone marrow or peripheral blood stem-cell transplants from related donors in adult patients with hematologic malignancies after myeloablative conditioning regimen, *Blood*, 2007;109:1322–30.

Index

A

B

C

D

G

H

I

J

K

L

M

N

O

P

Q

R

S

T

U

V

W

Y

Z